YOU'VE LOST WEIGHT!

THE EASY GUIDE TO RECEIVING THIS COMPLIMENT EVERY DAY

AF526937

DR SARITA DAVARE

SANJEEV KAPOOR

with

RITA D'SOUZA

Popular Prakashan

www.popularprakashan.com

Published by Harsha Bhatkal for
POPULAR PRAKASHAN PVT. LTD.
301, Mahalaxmi Chambers
22, Bhulabhai Desai Road
Mumbai–400 026
www.popularprakashan.com

© 2018 Sarita Davare
© 2018 Sanjeev Kapoor
First Published 2018

(4489)
ISBN: 978-81-7991-930-9

DISCLAIMER
The conclusions, beliefs and opinions expressed in this book, do not aim to diagnose, treat or prevent any illness, or condition, or guarantee any kind of weight loss whatsoever. The information provided in this book is intended as a guide only, and not as a substitute for advice from a registered physician, or any other qualified healthcare professional. The implementation of the diets mentioned in the book (whether in part or in whole) is entirely at your own risk and responsibility. You are advised to consult your physician before starting on The Live Well Diet.

WORLD RIGHTS RESERVED. The contents - all recipes, photographs and drawings are original and copyrighted. No portion of this book shall be reproduced, stored in a retrieval system or transmitted by any means, electronic, mechanical, photocopying, recording or otherwise, without the written permission of the author and the publisher.

Book Cover: Lantern Communications
Design: Anjali Sawant
Illustrations: Prabhakar Wairkar
Dr Davare's Photo: Veena Gokhale

Printed in India
by Saurabh Printers (P) Ltd.
Plot No. 67 A-68, Ecotech, Ext. I
Kasna, Greater Noida-201306 (U.P)

CONTENTS

SECTION III
Recipes

BREAKFAST

SOUPS

SALADS

SNACKS

MAIN DISHES - VEGETABLES

Author's Note: Dr Sarita Davare

You long to hear the words, "You've lost weight!" Especially if you have been trying for a long time to reduce your weight to what you think it should be. And when you hear someone utter that phrase with surprise and delight in their voice, you are over the moon with joy and a feeling of accomplishment. Suddenly, you will begin to walk taller and your shoulders, usually hunched in self-consciousness, straighten up; you feel confident, your smile gets wider, your face begins to glow and your eyes shine with happiness. In fact, the whole world seems to have become a better, brighter place.

I have watched many patients change before my eyes from individuals who were beaten down and despondent because of their excess weight and health problems, to bright, confident persons who appear to have got a new lease of life once they have lost weight. The transformation, I hasten to add, does not come overnight, and involves commitment, discipline, and changes in habits and lifestyle. For some, the process is easier than for others, but experience has shown that a genuine desire to achieve one's goals, a positive attitude and a holistic tried-and-tested plan, go a long way to remove the obstacles, both self-created and external, on the path to success and a life lived well.

This book shares the knowledge I have gained over the years of how to lose weight and live a healthy, happy life at the same time. My first book, *The Live Well Diet,* gives necessary and basic information to achieve weight loss and a healthy life. This book goes one step further and gives you strategies of how to acquire habits to achieve weight loss and how to counteract the impulses that prompt you to make excuses to avoid diets. It is a practical guide to achieving a well-balanced life with adequate and appropriate nutrition, physical activity, sleep and relaxation. In short, a diet and way of life that will help you to live well and to hear the words, "You've lost weight!" together with the phrase, "You look so good!" again and again.

For many of us, unfortunately, the word 'diet' is an unpleasant word. It is filled with all kinds of negative connotations like restrictions, lack of freedom, limited choice, endless suffering, suppression, pain, guilt, unsatisfied cravings, shame, pressure, starvation, and hunger. But worst of all, it seems to imply tasteless, bland and boring food.

Our natural reaction is to avoid going on a diet at all cost. We put it off and shy away from any restrictions recommended. We wriggle out of the commitment to healthier eating habits, no matter the urgency and imperative. We convince ourselves of the very good reasons why the dreaded diet should be postponed, or better still, cancelled forever.

Some of us, however, begin a diet with great enthusiasm and will power. Then gradually as boredom sets in and our resolve weakens, we look for ways out, and gradually let the diet fade to a complete stop. Only to get a rude awakening in the form of a health crisis, an unflattering image in a mirror or photograph, or a blunt comment. Then, of course, we start all over again.

The battle of the diets is one that is enacted by people of all ages all over the world. Today, there is a very real crisis of increasing obesity and lifestyle disease. This may seem at odds with the amount and variety of food choices available to us, including many healthy packaged foods. So how is one to cope with the need to make wise food choices with the demands of a very hectic modern lifestyle, and still come out a healthy, balanced individual who is living well and looking good too?

The answer is the Live Well Diet, which is more than just another diet. It is a way of life which is liberating: it offers a variety of food choices; it is very flexible with many options to adapt to life's many surprises, and yes, it prescribes delicious food that will both energise you, keep your body functioning optimally and help you to achieve your goal of losing weight and looking good.

My first book, *The Live Well Diet*, describes in great detail all the features of the diet. It explains the science behind the programme, and the changes you need to make to lead an active, healthy life. The diet is based on a few basic principles that are as simple as A, B and C. And that is what it is all about: 3 basic rotating food plans–A, B and C–which you choose based on your situation and needs. No boredom, no pressure, no exotic foods—rather, an intelligent set of flexible plans based on the way the human body absorbs, stores and burns energy from the food that we consume.

And it goes one step further. Built into the programme is the understanding of the human mind and will, and most importantly, the difficulty experienced in changing the habits of a lifetime, and the very real conflicts that confront every dieter, no matter how resolute, that prevent him or her from staying the course and achieving health goals. In this second book you will find tips and techniques to change old lifestyle and food habits and develop new ones that will ensure you eat well and live your best life.

The programme also recognises the compulsions and impulses of the yo-yo dieter, the slow-starter, the workaholic, the couch potato and many otherwise reasonable and rational individuals who suffer from a bad case of what I call 'Excusitis'. It is a state of mind or feeling that manifests itself whenever one is confronted with a diet plan, and which can afflict a person in a number of health-sabotaging ways. So tight is its hold, that it needs thoughtful, preventive measures and strong motivation to control and eradicate it completely.

In other words, Excusitis is a condition that affects the mind, prompting one to find a variety of excuses or 'good reasons' not to begin or stay on a diet, or engage in any physical activity that will lead to obvious health benefits. The reasons given are what one may call 'lame excuses', but they are very real to the person who is making them. The excuses stem from a very real apprehension about coping with, or a strong resistance to, changing the habits of an established lifestyle. As you will see, the Live Well Diet is the right prescription to prevent the onset of Excusitis, fight the symptoms and cure one of its harmful effects.

This diet is the result of many years of my research and practice, observing and treating patients with serious health problems who are reluctant or unable to make the changes required, even if they are in their own best interest. I have realised that it is the mind as well the body that has to be healed. Which is why I devised a holistic plan based on human nature and physiology. The diet is, therefore, varied and practical, yet with the desired impact on the body's metabolism, resulting in weight loss and overall improved health. In addition to the diet plans, there is an emphasis on good lifestyle habits—regular exercise, adequate sleep and relaxation to ensure a better quality of life.

I strongly recommend that you consult your physician before starting this or any other diet. This is particularly important if you are pregnant or menopausal; or if you are being treated for medical conditions such as diabetes, thyroid problems, high blood pressure, cardiac disease, psychological disorders or childhood obesity. Regular check-ups and a complete body profile are necessary to ensure your diet plan and programme are suited to your physical and mental well-being.

The diet plans themselves are full of exciting options that are suitable for the entire family who may not even suspect that they are being served 'diet food'. In addition, recipes by Master Chef Sanjeev Kapoor help you to live and eat really well, with enough delicious choices so you never have to suffer a moment's regret or give you any excuse to cheat!

Remember, living well is about caring for your mind and body by eating food that is nourishing, and engaging in activities that strengthen your body and calm your mind. So, begin by creating good eating and exercise habits, immunize yourself against Excusitis, and embrace a life of good health and satisfaction. You will then find you are receiving many compliments and congratulations, and your effort will be worth it.

Acknowledgements: Dr Sarita Davare

There are many people without whose help, active support and encouragement this book would never have seen the light of day. Over the years, I have forged a bond with several patients. My life is enriched by their friendship, loyalty and trust. My appreciation for their support knows no bounds.

My entire team at the Pain and Weight Management Clinic works tirelessly and with great dedication for the well-being of patients. I am very proud of them and appreciate their commitment. There are many doctors and medical professionals who have mentored, inspired and encouraged me with their advice and good wishes throughout my career.

My family has stood by me throughout and helped me achieve my dreams and goals. I am who I am because of their love and blessings.

I would like to especially thank Master Chef Sanjeev Kapoor, who encouraged me to write my books so that many more people could benefit from the Live Well Diet. He has also developed recipes that will come alive in your kitchen and support your resolution to choose a healthy lifestyle.

My special thanks to Harsha Bhatkal, my publisher, who has enthusiastically supported this book from the very beginning. Thanks to Vikram Sathaye for coming up with a very apt title.

I am very grateful to Rita D'Souza for helping me to put my knowledge and experience into words, and Swapna Shinde, Armaity Motafram and Anjali Sawant at Popular Prakashan who have put a lot of energy into preparing this book.

Author's Note: Sanjeev Kapoor

Living well can mean different things to different people–from owning a lavish apartment in a posh locality or the latest gadget, to treating yourself at a super fine-dine restaurant or taking a holiday every now and then! However, I would like to suggest that living well is quite an art and much more than that—it has less to do with the health of one's bank balance, and much more to do with the state of one's health–physical, mental and emotional.

To live well is to enjoy the freedom of being able to walk, and even run, no matter what your age, to climb a flight of stairs without getting out of breath, to eat a good meal without feeling any discomfort or ill effects–all tensions at bay. Besides this, you also know that you're living well when you:

- Wake up refreshed in the morning
- Take interest in doing good to others as well as contributing to their wellness
- Live in the moment
- Are confident and have an optimistic approach to life
- Are alert, grateful and engaged in life
- Constantly turn obstacles into opportunities

The glow of one's skin and the spring in one's step is more evidence of truly living well than any manifestation of wealth. Thus, it can be rightly said that the difference between 'living well' and 'just living' is pretty much similar to preparing a meal when you're hungry–preparing a dish with whatever is at hand without taking the taste, nutrition, visual appeal, etc. into consideration, versus preparing the same dish by putting your heart and soul into it to create a complete experience. Health is surely wealth, but in today's jet-set age, many of us take our bodies and well-being for granted.

Anything in excess is always harmful! So, one of the things that's a sure sign of not living well is being over or underweight. It can have serious and long-term effects on our physical and mental well-being. The market is full of solutions that promise instant results for your weight and ultimately mental bliss. But there are very few that have been tried and tested and become a way of life for countless people.

The Live Well Diet is one such solution, and Alyona and I, along with other family members and friends, are the proof of its efficacy. We are really happy about incorporating the diet and its principles in our lives, and it is no longer a diet but a way of being. We no longer have to agonise over the food choices we make as we know that we have the tools and knowledge to cope with any situation. My profession requires a lot of travelling, and with this diet, I find it perfectly comfortable to maintain my eating habits within the parameters prescribed. Also, it is a boon, as I know for sure that it does not have serious side effects. I have learnt to be proactive and to plan, to recover from a lapse and move forward without looking back. My exercise regimes complement my food habits and I have structured my life to allow me to make the right choices and do what is necessary to really and truly 'live well'.

Dr. Sarita Davare's Live Well Diet is a holistic approach to leading a fit, healthy and balanced life. Being convinced of the ideas, I felt compelled to contribute, and develop recipes based on the principles and recommendations on which the diet is based. I offer these recipes to you so that you too can benefit from making the right choices without fear of a diet that is bland or boring. There is plenty of variety, and the options are both tasty and nutritious, so taste is not sacrificed at the altar of good health. You will find it is easy to make healthy eating a part of your life when you can always have a plate of deliciousness in front of you.

But, it all begins with wanting to make a change and to making the right choices. I hope that this book will help you on your journey towards wellness, and that the change will be positive, liberating and full of opportunities. Most of all, I wish you 'live well' each day of your life, and that you begin to often hear those magic words, "You've lost weight!"

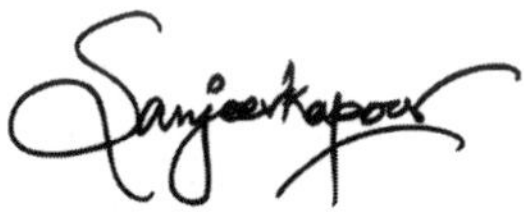

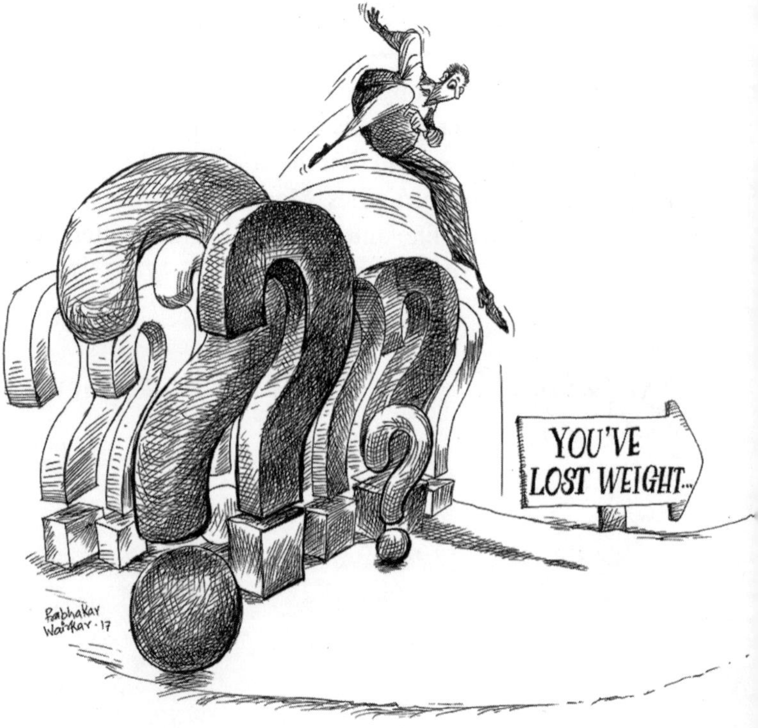
YOU'VE
LOST WEIGHT...
Prabhakar
Wadkar · 17

SECTION I

1

Meet The Live Well Diet

The secret to living well is encapsulated in the old saying, "a healthy mind in a healthy body". Positive thinking, a must do-can-do spirit, a calm and relaxed disposition, good self esteem, and balanced, nutritious, regular eating habits are what it takes to lead a personal life of physical and mental well-being. In short, a holistic and practical approach to one's lifestyle and personal habits. The Live Well Diet is a practical guide to achieving a well-balanced life with adequate and appropriate nutrition. It also provides tips to change the habits of a lifetime that prevent one from living a comfortable life of good health. Once you have got to know and understand the diet it will become a trusted and faithful companion that will steer you through the challenges you face to achieve your health goals.

The diet is based on experience and knowledge of how the body's metabolism functions. Metabolism, or the process of converting the food we eat into energy, determines one's state of health and well-being: the more efficient one's metabolism, the better one's general state of health.

There are many factors that cause metabolism to function at an optimum rate, and many that slow it down to the point where it begins to have a negative impact on one's weight and overall health. The Live Well Diet recognises that to function optimally, a varied, rotating eating plan, ample water and liquid nourishment, regular physical activity and enough sleep, encourage the body to burn energy from the food consumed in an efficient way.

A High-Protein, High-Fibre Diet: The emphasis is on foods that provide plenty of good quality protein and complex carbohydrates that give the body energy and help to build muscle rather than excess fat. Fish, chicken, lentils, legumes and pulses, together with fibre-rich vegetables, fruit and whole grains (sorghum/jowar, oats/jai, millets/nachni, bajra) form the basis of the diet. Foods high in fat (oil, butter, ghee), sugar (including sugary fruit), starch, and salt are to be consumed very sparingly.

A, B and C Diet Plans: The diet consists of 3 rotating daily eating plans (3 main meals and 3 to 4 small meals) to be followed in a specific order to stimulate the body's metabolic system.

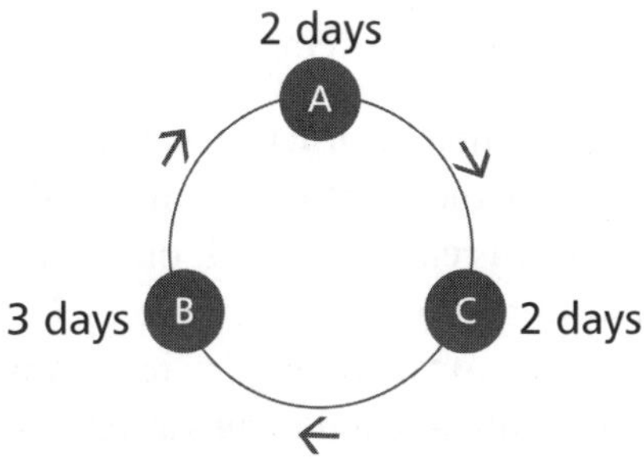

Plan A (All Foods Plan) has a variety of foods and is perfect for holidays or weekends when one can indulge in one's favourite foods. For that very reason, Plan A must invariably be followed by **Plan C (Control Plan)**, that is a high-protein, low-carbohydrate plan, which will steer one back on track and help the body to burn the extra energy consumed the previous day. **Plan B (Basic Plan)** anchors the diet in a regular and balanced eating programme, that prescribes high-fibre mainly vegetarian foods, that can form the basis of any long-term diet as well. The recommended weekly diet schedule is 2 days of Plan A, 3 days of Plan B and 2 days of Plan C.

Water: Drinking plenty of water—at least 3 to 4 litres a day, 2 of which are flavoured with lime juice—helps to flush the system of toxins and excess fat stored, stimulates the metabolism and hydrates the body.

Other healthy beverages like vegetable juices, coconut water and buttermilk, provide essential nutrients and encourage metabolic activity.

Exercise: A diet by itself will yield good results, but to be truly effective, it is necessary to engage in regular age and health-appropriate physical activity. Daily basic yoga breathing exercises and stretches, plus 45 minutes of brisk walking, or an hour at the gym, are essential to give the whole body, particularly the metabolic system, a good work out.

Relaxation: A calm mind in an active body is the secret to living well. Stress is one of the most common modern afflictions—no one escapes it. To really live well, one has to combat and prevent stress from taking over one's life by carving out time from busy schedules to relax, engage in a satisfying activity, meditate or just be still. A good night's sleep is also invaluable: besides refreshing the mind and body, sleep has a positive effect on the metabolism.

Moderation and Balance: Too much or too little of anything is bound to have negative consequences. And that applies to food, water, exercise, sleep and stress. Too little food can lead to conditions such as anorexia, and too much food can result in obesity; too little water can lead to dehydration and an impaired metabolic system, and too much water may lead to water intoxication with dangerously low sodium levels in the blood; too much exercise can lead to exercise addiction and fatigue; and too little exercise with a sedentary lifestyle can lead to weight gain and flabby muscles; too little sleep can lead to stress and other nervous conditions, and too much in turn takes its toll on one's mental and physical well-being. Balance and moderation, therefore, are essential for healthy living and they are one of the founding principles of the Live Well Diet.

Flexibility: The best features of the diet are its flexibility and adaptability. It provides for both proactive as well as corrective measures for situations that crop up in everyday life that sabotage a rigid eating plan. Weddings, parties, travel, holidays, fun weekends or just plain off days, are all catered for in the programme. Switching from one plan to another, making up for a heavy meal, or anticipating a day off the plan are all possible, and recommended, so that overall balance and regularity are maintained. On-the-spot solutions for tricky situations like a sudden attack of hunger pangs are also prescribed, so one never need feel guilty or endanger the entire programme by over-indulgence provoked by a rumbling tummy.

Variety: Boredom is the enemy of diets. Recognising this fact, the rotating diet plans prescribed provide a variety and assortment of foods so meals are always appetising and full of flavour. Recipes developed by Master Chef Sanjeev Kapoor provide many ideas to make your meals more interesting, so you may really never feel you are on a diet at all.

Accessibility: Many diets and health programmes fail because their demands are either too expensive or too specific, acting as stumbling blocks to their full implementation. The foods prescribed here are everyday basic dishes based on easily available ingredients that can be turned into delicious meals. No special equipment is required to exercise either—just a brisk walk and a few breathing and stretching exercises every day.

10 Mantras to Live Well

1. **Eat Right:** Foods that are rich in fibre, protein, minerals and vitamins essential for good health and an active metabolism.
2. **Eat Often:** 3 main meals and 3-4 small meals a day, including healthy beverages and snacks.
3. **Eat Just Enough:** Portion size is an important and practical way of regulating how much you eat.
4. **Drink Plenty of Water and Beverages:** You need at least 3 to 4 litres of water a day, as well as vegetable and fruit juices to hydrate, detoxify and nourish your system.
5. **Pamper Your Taste Buds:** Eat well, and with pleasure, the variety of foods offered by the A, B and C diet plans.
6. **Boost Your Metabolism:** Eat the right foods in the right combination, detoxify your system with water and get active to keep your metabolism ticking.
7. **Stay on Track:** Use the flexible diet plans to anticipate a challenging diet situation, or to make up for a lapse in your scheduled plan. Once you have achieved your target or desired weight, remember to stay within 2 kg. of that weight.
8. **Exercise:** A few minutes of yoga and breathing exercises, a brisk walk for 45 minutes a day and simple stretching exercises are all you need to keep your body fit and your metabolism active.
9. **Relax and Sleep:** 7 hours of sleep a day with a few minutes of meditation, and an engaging hobby will ensure a relaxed and positive frame of mind and good mental health.
10. **Record Your Progress:** Consult your physician before you begin the diet and have a complete body profile test done. Keep track of your body weight and measurements, and health records, and revel in the changes. Make sure you do a complete body profile at least once a year.

From My Case Files

A young woman walked into my clinic a few months ago. She was an overweight mother struggling to cope with the demands of two active young children when all she wanted to do was sleep. She had been diagnosed as suffering from hypersomnia, or too much sleep, perhaps as a result of her obesity—she weighed 84 kg. After consulting with me, she decided to go on the Live Well Diet and soon managed to lose 14 kg. Her sleep habits changed and she began to feel positive and more active. She stayed that way for 3 years, all the while following the diet, exercise and relaxation plans that had become a part of her lifestyle.

Unfortunately, due to a difficult personal situation, she underwent a great deal of stress that took its toll on her mental and physical well-being. She abandoned her diet, as a result of which her weight shot up to 90 kg, her body feeling heavy and bloated due to fluid retention and oedema. She soon realised that the only way out of her situation was to go back to the basic principles of the diet. She made the tough decision to follow the diet plans rigorously and started her daily walks and yoga.

Soon, she began to lose weight, sleep better, recover her peace of mind and have a more positive outlook on life. Once she reached her target weight she was determined to maintain the lifestyle changes that had benefited her mentally and physically, and which had given her the strength and ability to overcome any challenges that would come her way.

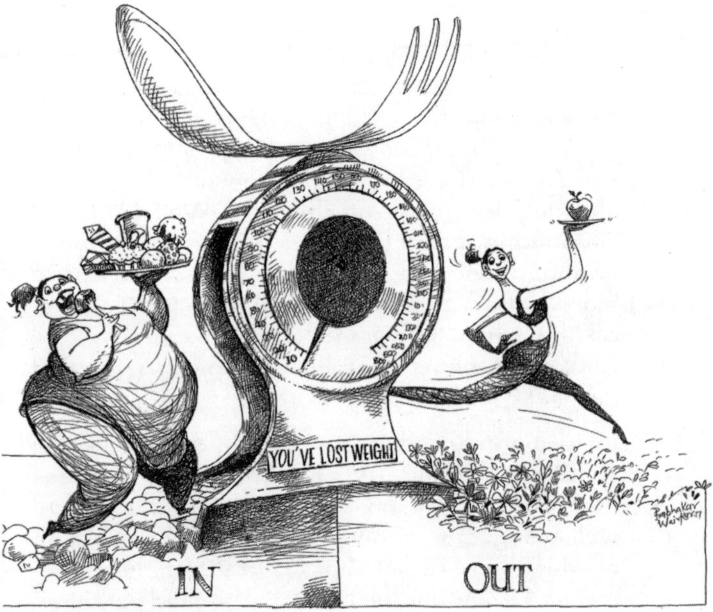
YOU'VE LOST WEIGHT
IN
OUT

2

Why You Need The Live Well Diet

A variety of patients from all walks of life, of different ages and cultural backgrounds, visit my clinic every day. There is the middle-aged man suffering from chronic obesity who has been referred to me by a cardiologist; another gentleman who has tried several health clinics and gyms to lose weight and who wants to try one more–'kar ke dekhenge' is his philosophy. Then, there is the woman who has been sent to my clinic by her husband who wants a slimmer wife. Another woman has been referred to my clinic by her gynaecologist as she has trouble conceiving a child because she is overweight. Young women and men who want to have the svelte and toned-up bodies like their celebrity heroes or heroines are common visitors to my clinic. The most urgent and desperate requests come from bridegrooms and brides-to-be who want to look slim and gorgeous on their wedding day.

Quick fixes don't work. Persevere! When you feel like giving up, think about why you started!

For most of these patients, weight loss is a quick fix to an immediate problem and not a lifestyle choice. Which is why their efforts are sporadic and temporary and doomed to fail. The ones who succeed are those who persevere, and change their eating and exercise habits so they can truly live a healthy life.

Given below are some reasons you may want to follow the Live Well Diet for a lifetime of good health.

You weigh more than you should or want to.

Scales, they say, do not lie; neither do measuring tapes or mirrors. There are height-weight charts easily available to let you know if your weight is within the ideal range for your gender and height (page 312).

Waist measurements are also an easy way to let you know if you are overweight. For men it is a waist measurement of more than 90 cm (35 inches), and for women, more than 80 cm (30.5 inches). Besides, there are enough visual clues that your mirror will give you, and your clothes that may have become too small for you will indicate whether you are piling on the kilos and inches. If nothing else, an uninhibited relative or dear friend will whisper the awful truth in your ear, or snatch away that bar of chocolate just as you are about to take a bite.

You have health problems like diabetes, high blood pressure, breathlessness, and cardio-vascular or thyroid disease.

You may not be overweight, but still suffer from one or more of the lifestyle diseases that have become so common these days. Most of these diseases, however, are linked to obesity or excess body weight. They can be treated partially by changes in your lifestyle and diet.

You just don't feel bright and energetic.

This may be because your metabolism is sluggish or slow, and your body is not able to burn the energy consumed through food in an optimum way. You, therefore, feel tired and listless, suffer from headaches and have a poor appetite. Other symptoms of a sluggish metabolism include acidity, bloating and gradual weight gain.

Your eating habits are irregular and your diet is too unbalanced for a healthy life.

You are not able to maintain regular eating habits and a nutritionally balanced diet—a condition that will eventually lead to health problems. Regulating your food and adding exercise to your daily routine will keep you fit and improve the quality of your life.

You have an emotional dependence on food.

You live to eat and find it hard to control your eating habits and appetite. You consciously, or unconsciously, look at food as the solution to your emotional problems and allow food to control your life. Your dependence on food can become life-threatening if not taken in hand and you do not regulate your eating.

You want to live well.

You have very few eating problems and your health is good, but you want to live a better life. All those compliments about how slim you look are a bonus!

From My Case Files

It came as a shock to this young woman when she realised her dress size had increased to XXL. Her weight had gradually increased over the years and she found she now had to buy clothes designed for larger women. She came to me for help to lose weight but was apprehensive about not following the diet plans. She made a decision to give it a try and found that she began to lose weight. She grew more confident as her weight as well as her dress sizes dropped. She now weighs 57 kg having lost 25 kilos, and her dress size has gone from XXL to M. So happy is she with the results that she has made living well a habit.

Your Diet And You

So you know you need to or want to diet, but the most common reaction to going on a diet is not to! The reasons or excuses are plenty and varied, and sometimes very creative. Most dieters have 'been there, done that', and behind all the enthusiasm born out of desperation lies a cynicism which almost dares the diet to succeed! How you perceive a diet determines how well you will succeed in changing your eating habits and your lifestyle.

There are so many diets out there to choose from and you have probably tried quite a few yourself. There are those based on single ingredients like the boiled egg diet; the blood type diet; crash diets; soup and juice diets; the carbohydrate-rich diet; the paleo diet; the keto diet; and many different high-fat and high-protein diets. There seem to be diets based on every type of personality and every type of food.

The Live Well Diet is reasonable, sustainable and smart.

The truth is that most diets fail because they make too many demands, are too restrictive and are difficult to follow on a long-term basis. Most diets, again, offer quick-fix options that may help you to lose weight in the short term, but which cannot be sustained over a lifetime. This is where the Live Well Diet differs from most other diets. It is a diet and a way of life that is reasonable, sustainable and smart, as it incorporates a variety of food choices, is practical and can be followed by people of all ages.

The unique and best aspect of the diet is that it is based on experience and the study of the psychology of a great number of patients with reference to their eating habits and relationship to food. It takes into consideration various reactions that have been reported and descriptions of past relationships with diets that many have experienced. It prescribes a varied practical eating plan and way of life to overcome most negative experiences and perceptions.

Here are some ways people view their experiences with diets and the restrictions placed upon them. You can change that perception to a more supportive one and feel the difference. For every negative perception that you may have, there is another that is positive and helpful. It all depends on your point of view!

A series of obstacles *to be surmounted involving hard work, sweat and strain—the rocky road to success.*

A bitter pill *or a series of bitter pills I have to swallow–so I will eventually be healthy.*

An unfair punishment *for a genetic mishap–poor me! Fate played a cruel trick on me and loaded me with fat genes for which I have to pay a terrible price.*

A life sentence*–the severe punishment for my past sins of overeating and leading a lazy life.*

A trap *or a vice whose grip I can't get out of or escape without the severest consequences.*

A minefield t*hat I have to negotiate with skill and care or it will blow up in my face.*

An overwhelming task *at which I am guaranteed to fail.*

A challenge *for which I must roll up my sleeves and prepare to meet head on.*

Don't be surprised if you have ticked several or all the negative statements! You are in the company of many who have been in a similar position. These negative perceptions are understandable, particularly if you have been a serial dieter and experienced many life-crippling diets, or tried too hard to achieve too much in too short a time. As with other relationships, it will be some time before you trust the diet and yourself again.

But, I can assure you, once you experience the freedom and choices the Live Well Diet offers, you will realise that far from being the enemy, it can become your friend. It is designed to be a caring and nurturing support system providing you with all the help you need to ensure that you enjoy a healthy and satisfied life. Restrictions there are, but the diet provides enough unrestricted and delicious foods so you need never feel deprived or depressed. There are also proactive and recovery strategies, so any situations that threaten to sabotage your diet are dealt with promptly and smartly.

TURN YOUR LIFE AROUND

Let the Live Well Diet change from being

an enemy ➔ a caring friend
a series of obstacles ➔ a helping hand
a bitter pill ➔ a delicious remedy
an unfair punishment ➔ a just reward
a life sentence ➔ a lifetime of wellness
a trap ➔ freedom
a minefield ➔ stepping stones
an overwhelming task ➔ small steps leading to success
a challenge ➔ an opportunity

From My Case Files

A young married woman, aged 29, was very distressed as she was very overweight and when tested had discovered that her prolactin levels were very high—76 ng/ml! Normal prolactin levels for women who are not pregnant are below 25 ng/ml (nanograms per milliliter). She told me that she had put on 18 kg after her marriage, and weighed 82 kg when she came to consult me. She also suffered from severe headaches, one of the common symptoms of excess prolactin. She began the Live Well Diet, which she followed religiously for several months. She now weighs 62 kg, and best of all, her prolactin levels at 20mg/ml have dropped to normal levels. The most rewarding fact is that she achieved this without any medication, only by changing her food habits and lifestyle.

Yes, You Can!

I am constantly amazed at the variety of reasons I have heard from patients about why they cannot, or find it difficult to, go on a diet. One of the most common statements I have heard is, "I will never be able to stick to a diet–I do not have the will power." There are others who have a very carefree attitude believing that "nothing will happen to me if I continue with my present way of life". As I have often seen, this is potentially a very dangerous attitude that can lead to grave consequences in the form of serious medical conditions. Still others believe that diets in general are too restrictive requiring all of one's mental resources to follow the recommendations. When I hear that I always ask the question, "Why do you want to diet at all?"

Conversations with my clients often go something like this:

Me : I have the ideal diet for you.

Patient : I will never be able to stick to a diet.

Me : Why do you think that?

Patient : I have tried many diets and I have always failed. I don't even last a week. Once I managed to do it for a month but then I gave up.

Me : So, why do you want to diet?

Patient : Because my doctor says I am overweight.

Me : But why do YOU want to diet?

Patient : Because my wife says I must do something about how I look.

Me : What do you mean?

Patient : See - I have a paunch and my shirt is so tight. I also have a double chin which makes my face look fat.

Me : And?

Patient : I can't bend down easily to put on my shoes. I get breathless when I walk or climb stairs.

Me : Yes, and...?

Patient : And I am so uncomfortable I can't even sleep well at night.

Me : Is that why you want to diet then?

Patient : I suppose so.

Me : So, if you are so uncomfortable and unhappy about how you look and everyone thinks you should diet, what's the problem—why can't you follow a diet?

Patient : I don't know...I just can't!

Me : Yes, you can!

Somewhere inside you know that you need to change your lifestyle; not just because your doctor, or your spouse or your friends tell you to, but because you feel uncomfortable and uneasy. However, you are just not mentally motivated enough to do anything about it.

Motivation is the key to success in any venture. If you want something badly enough you will make it happen. Giving up or avoidance is such an easy way out. In these days of instant gratification and quick-fix solutions, it may appear to be futile to struggle long and hard to achieve anything worthwhile, including one's own good health.

The first step on the path to living well is a strong desire to change, and the fervent belief that you have the will and the strength to stay the course.

The Live Well Diet is the answer for anyone who knows what needs to be done, but is finding it difficult to change, or reluctant to live by the restrictions and discipline a diet usually demands. It is designed to provide variety and flexibility within a framework that gives you the freedom to adapt the diet to every situation and make appropriate choices. So if you follow the Live Well Diet plans, yes, you certainly can and will begin to live well. And as you do, see those extra kilos and inches slowly slip away, and bask in the compliments that come your way.

"In order to succeed, we must first believe that we can."

— Nikos Kazantzakis

Take the First Steps to a Healthier Happier You!

1. Shrug off the inertia
2. Dispel those doubts
3. Get a grip over your wavering thoughts
4. Tell yourself, "enough is enough" with the old unhealthy lifestyle
5. Start NOW!

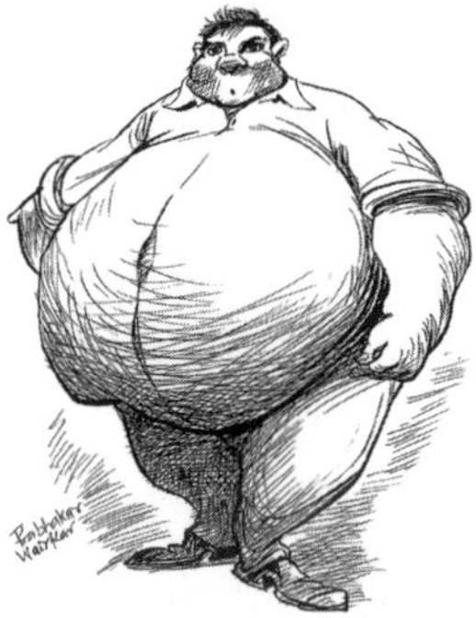

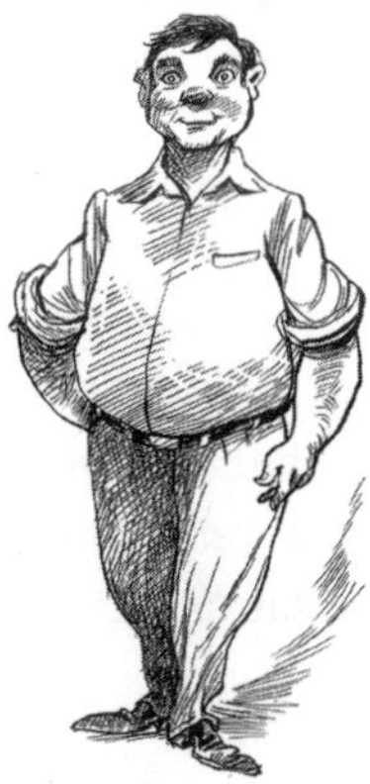

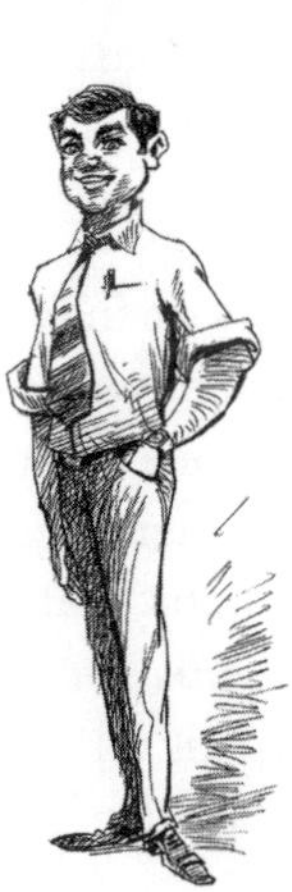

3

Habits—Paths Well-Travelled

"Motivation is what gets you started. Habit is what keeps you going."

— Jim Ryun

So, why is it so difficult to change? Especially when you desperately want to; and logic, common sense, your doctor, your medical reports, your best friend and your body all tell you that you need to. Perhaps it is because you have developed over the years those stubborn, unshakeable companions—habits!

A habit is an automatic, almost unconscious, response to a situation: a behaviour that has been learned and formed over a long period of time, performing the same action and responding to the same situation in the same way.

Habits are what make us who we are. How we dress, how we eat, how we work; what time we rise and what time we go to bed; whether we can't eat toast without butter or drink tea without milk; how loud or soft we like our music; and the list goes on.

Most habits are formed early on in life, and once formed can be difficult to change. Research has shown that there is a scientific reason for it—repeated actions forge a neurological pathway in the brain that gets more ingrained every time the action is performed. If a particular habit makes you feel good, or leads to what you consider to be positive results, you are very likely going to repeat it. The repetition reinforces the behaviour or action, and the habit gets further ingrained or set. Once the neurological pathway has been established, it can be difficult to overwrite or circumnavigate it with a different path. It requires perseverance, determination and a conscious effort to change an established habit, particularly one that is undesirable or harmful.

"First we make our habits, then our habits make us."

— Charles C. Noble

But do not despair—it IS possible to change a well-established way of eating and living, and the Live Well Diet gives you all the tools and techniques to make the desirable changes in your life happen.

How habits are made

A situation acts as a trigger or cue to which you respond in a certain way every time (habitual response); and as you complete the action you feel a sense of satisfaction for having responded in that way and are pleased with the results of the response. Therefore, you respond to the trigger or cue in the same way every time, thus creating a habit. Most habits are unconscious acts, where actions are not preplanned or thought about, but merely reactions to given situations. A habit can be good or bad—it all depends on the positive or negative outcome of a habitual action. Here are some examples:

1. **Cue or trigger:** Your mobile beeps.

   Habitual automatic response: You immediately check your mobile.
   Reward or satisfaction: You get to know at once who called or sent a message and its contents.

2. **Cue or trigger:** You see a spoon with jam or pickle clinging to it on your dining table or kitchen counter.

   Habitual automatic response: You pick up and lick the spoon.

Reward or satisfaction: The taste of the jam or pickle, and the belief built over time that you are not letting anything go to waste!

3. **Cue or trigger:** You enter your home.

   Habitual automatic response: You take off your shoes just inside the door.

   Reward or satisfaction: You are making sure you do not bring dirt into your clean home.

4. **Cue or trigger:** You are watching television.

   Habitual automatic response: You eat a snack while you watch: a packet of wafers, a bowl of popcorn or a plate of onion bhajji.

   Reward or satisfaction: Dual enjoyment of the food and entertainment—keeping your mouth and your mind busy.

The Circle of Habit Formation

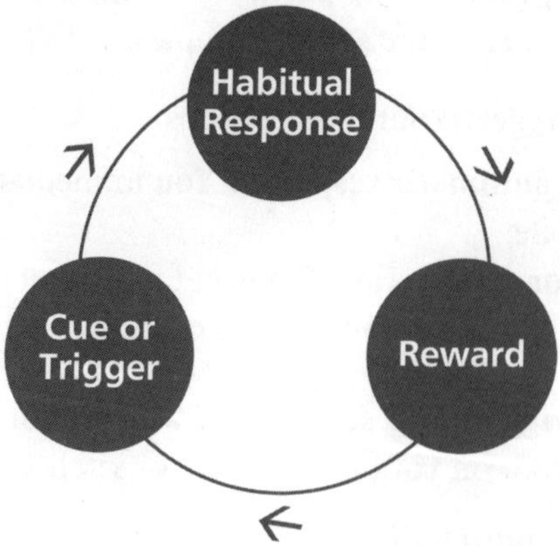

If you want to change a habit, you must first change the habitual or automatic response to a cue or trigger; and then replace the habitual response with one that is desirable and helpful. In addition, expect a different reward or satisfaction from the new habit that is more desirable than the previous one.

"Habits are at first cobwebs, then cables."

— Spanish Proverb

From My Case Files

I have a very loyal patient, a 57-year old woman, who has immense faith in the Live Well Diet that she has been following for several years.

Recently, she underwent tests for suspected osteoporosis and surprised her doctor with the results: her Vitamins D3 and B12 levels, usually very low in patients suffering from osteoporosis, were completely normal. A result, no doubt, of her controlled eating habits and faithfulness to the diet.

Changes You Believe In

Good habits and bad habits

As with any behaviour, there are those actions that will bring positive or beneficial results, and those actions that will have negative or harmful consequences. The problem arises when one finds it difficult to decide which habits are serving us well and which are actually hurting us. Some habits are easy to label good or bad but others may be a little difficult to identify as they have become so much a part of our lives and who we are. By the time you finish reading this book you will be able to identify those habits that you need to keep and those you will need to change if you want to live a life of good health.

The 5 Rs that will help you to change a habit

Changing a habitual response to one that is desirable will take some perseverance until that new response becomes automatic and habitual. And yes, it takes work and the progress may be slow, but the results in the end are lasting and worthwhile. Remember the saying, "sabr ka phal meetha hota hai." (the fruit of patience is always sweet).

There are 5 essential aids or steps to permanently changing a habit, and each one is as important as the others. They are: **recognition** or **realisation** of the habit that has to be changed; a mental and physical **readiness** to make the necessary changes; a new **routine** response to a cue or trigger so that the old habit is slowly replaced; **reminders** that will encourage the desirable response every time; and lastly, the **reward**—the satisfaction of having produced the desirable response to a situation, and its overall positive impact on your lifestyle and well-being.

RECOGNITION OR REALISATION

As with any situation that requires change, the first step is to identify what behaviours need to be changed, and why. This involves not just identification but also acceptance of the changes. To live well what you may need to change are behaviours and habits such as:

- poor food choices–too much junk or fattening food
- lack of physical activity
- overeating
- skipping meals
- not drinking enough water
- emotional eating
- not sleeping enough

The reasons to change may be many, but they will all involve a strong desire, and perhaps necessity, to live a better and healthier life.

READINESS

You know what has to change and the reasons or compulsions to make the change, but you may not be ready to make those changes mentally, physically or emotionally. Much as we would like to believe otherwise, change takes more than a strong will. As I often tell my patients, "Changing habits is simple, but not easy."

A strong motivation is an important factor in effecting long-lasting change: how committed and passionate you are to leading a different way of life will determine your success.

There are many situations that you come across, which tempt or encourage you to deviate from a chosen path. Preparing the physical environment around you by removing undesirable foods and stocking your kitchen with appropriate foods; or rescheduling your priorities to accommodate your exercise routine, require thoughtful planning and a mental preparedness to succeed in making the necessary changes.

A strong motivation is an important factor in effecting long-lasting change: how committed and passionate you are to leading a different way of life will determine your success.

Readiness also involves setting yourself achievable and reasonable goals. Nothing is worse than setting the bar for yourself so high that it is impossible to reach. Frustration at not being able to change may lead to stress, which in turn may only reinforce the undesirable habit. For example, if you decide to exercise every day and start by walking 6 km on the first day itself, you may do yourself harm, and the aches and pains you suffer will dissuade you from making another attempt, thus thwarting any chance of making the habit of exercising every day a reality.

ROUTINE

Nothing is more important than a routine to help you change. You need to repeat the same actions and make the same changes in your behaviour so you rewrite the pathways in your brain that formed your original habits. In other words, change the responses to the cues or triggers presented by a situation. You will have to make a conscious effort not to reach for that slab of chocolate after a meal, but to opt for a piece of fruit instead; to stop visiting the mithaiwalla on your way home from the market every Saturday; to set the alarm so you can wake up bright and early to get in your daily exercise; to drink that warm water with a squeeze of lime as you wake each day; and to go to bed at a reasonable time every night.

Soon, you will be on autopilot, navigating through difficult situations with the confidence that comes from well-ingrained unconscious responses to situations you are faced with.

Many of my patients start out by clutching on to the diet plans as though their lives depended on them (they very often do!), but soon they find they can figure out the appropriate response and choice of food without reference to any notes—they have learned and internalized the eating habits and food choices that enable them to achieve their goals.

Every small change you work into your daily routine and food choices will reinforce your new life-changing habits.

REMINDERS

You will be fooling yourself if you think you will be able to accomplish the necessary changes without any help. You will need the support of friends and family, as well as a number of techniques and tools that will nudge you gently towards changing the offending habit. Give your spouse, best friend or a person you trust the permission to remind you of your goals and keep you on track. Such a champion of change will snatch that laddoo from you; remind you to set your morning alarm; get rid of that packet of wafers hidden behind the TV; help you to choose the right dish in a restaurant; or accompany you on your walk.

A weekly or daily meal plan and a 'good food' list stuck on the refrigerator; mobile phone alarms to remind you to drink water or eat your snack; notes to yourself; a daily food diary; post-its with encouraging messages; a photograph of yourself in slimmer days; regular medical reports and weight checks are all ways to remind you of what is at stake, and the habits you need to acquire to achieve your goals.

REWARDS

Every effort needs reward and recognition, and so it is with changing your habits and way of life. Watching the needle on the scales begin to drop and the extra inches disappear should be reward enough. A fresher appearance, glowing skin, firmer body and well-toned muscles are some of the rewards you will bestow on yourself with your change in lifestyle. And there is much more—more energy, better medical reports, a feeling of mental and emotional well-being, a calmer more relaxed disposition, and more than anything else, a renewed self-confidence. Best of all you hear the words, "You've lost weight" often which boosts your self-confidence and encourages you to continue your effort to change your lifestyle.

Speaking of rewards, after sticking to your diet and doing your daily exercise don't reward yourself with junk food! Instead, give your self a non-edible treat such as a visit to a spa, or a theatre to watch a good movie.

And if you slip up and fall down at any one of the steps? Pick yourself up, remind yourself of your goal of healthy living, continue where you left off and just keep going. Don't give up!

The secret of change is to focus all of your energy not on fighting the old but on building the new.

— Socrates

SWEET SUCCESS

How I overcame my addiction to sweets.

RECOGNITION/REALISATION

I am overweight. I must give up my habit of eating sweets, especially after a meal.

READINESS

I empty my refrigerator, kitchen cabinets and drawers of all sweets, mithai, toffees and chocolate, including drawers in my desk and bedside table.

I buy fruit, dried dates and a small quantity of chikki to indulge my sweet tooth without any harmful effects.

I delete the apps and telephone numbers of pastry/mithai shops and ice cream parlours on my mobile phone as I know I might on impulse call 'just this once'.

ROUTINE

Instead of dessert, I eat a piece of fruit or dried fruit after my meal.

I carry a few pieces of chikki and dried fruit with me to cater to my cravings for something sweet.

REMINDER

I place a piece of fruit or dried fruit alongside my plate before I sit down to eat. I request my friends to support me when we go to a restaurant by reminding me that I should not order dessert.

I request my family and friends to refuse to accede to my requests to buy mithai, or to insist I try the new dessert.

REWARD

I gradually begin to lose my desire to eat sweets. I begin to lose weight and inches around my waist. I get into the habit of eating fruit or dried fruit instead of sweets.

Make a Habit of Living Well

"We are what we repeatedly do. Excellence then, is not an act, but a habit."

— Aristotle

Below is a list of some habits that will help you to lose weight and live well. These are broad suggestions, but you will have to break them down to make your own list of smaller habits that you need to acquire that will permanently change your relationship with food and the way you live. The list may seem overwhelming, but most of it involves planning a menu, stocking up on the right foods and fitting an exercise and relaxation plan into your schedule.

"Sometimes the smallest step in the right direction ends up being the biggest step of your life."

— Anonymous

The important thing is not to be overwhelmed by the list of changes you have to make, but take one step at a time and make small changes at first that will make a visible difference in your lifestyle, which in turn will encourage you to make more changes as you go along. Too quick and too many changes all at once can be disastrous and lead to frustration. However, you must keep your goal always in mind and make as many changes in your habits that you can cope with without completely giving up in frustration.

In my many years of practice, I have come across patients who prepare for a life of fitness with great enthusiasm. They buy trendy sports shoes, gym wear and water bottles. They begin by walking briskly the entire 6 km on the very first day. They are so exhausted by the end of it with muscle pain and cramps in their legs that they give up and decide never to exercise again!

Begin by walking a shorter distance at a slow speed, gradually increasing the speed and distance until you are able to complete the entire distance at a regular pace.

The same goes for your food choices. Crash dieting will end in the crashing of any motivation and success in your efforts to eat appropriately. Your diet should never be a desperate attempt to control your eating habits, but a systematic, programmed and controlled approach to food and eating.

Here is a list of habits that you will need to live well. Tick the ones you would like to focus on at the start and make the necessary changes. Incorporate other good food habits as you go along.

Food Habits

- Eat at regular times every day.
- Eat 3 larger and 3 to 4 small meals a day.
- Drink at least 4 litres of water in addition to other nutrition-rich beverages every day.
- Eat breakfast every day.
- Eat a variety of foods every day in a balanced way.
- Include more fresh fruits and vegetables in your diet.
- Eat at least one type of whole grain every day such as whole-wheat (gehun), oats (jai), sorghum (jowar), and pearl millet (bajra).
- Avoid, or very occasionally, eat foods that contain fat.
- Reduce your salt and sugar intake.
- Reduce or avoid alcohol intake.

Physical Activity

- Do some physical exercise or activity for a minimum of 30 minutes at least 5 times a week.
- Do stretching exercises such as yoga at least 3 times a week.

Leisure and Relaxation

- Engage in a hobby or relaxing pastime.
- Practice yoga or other relaxation or meditation techniques.
- Get at least 7 hours sleep every night.
- Avoid tobacco in any form.

Health Status

- Monitor your weight regularly.
- Take nutritional supplements.
- Have regular medical check-ups.
- Maintain a food and weight diary.

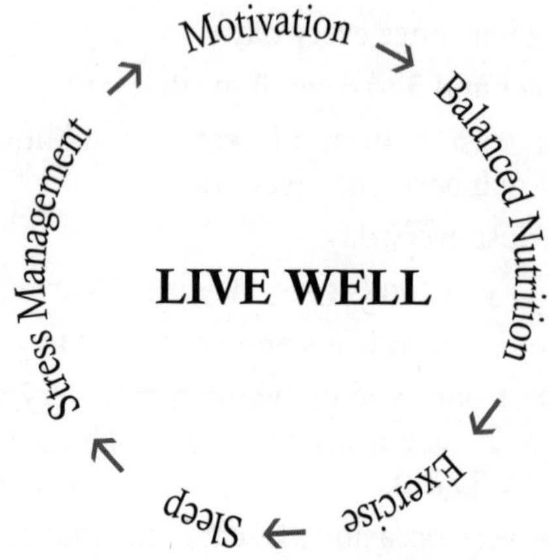

It takes 21 days to create a habit and 90 days to create a lifestyle! So take the first steps now!

4

Excusitis–The Worst Habit of All, and How to Beat it!

"Ninety-nine percent of failures come from people who have the habit of making excuses."

— George Washington Carver

You have cleaned out your kitchen cabinets of all unhealthy foods. You have stocked up on nutrient-rich and low-calorie edibles; your refrigerator is full of lean, green veggies, and luscious fruit; the new trainers are out of their box, and the track suit ready; the trendy slim water bottle is filled and chilling in the refrigerator, when suddenly…pfffft! Planning, preparation and resolve vanish in a flash. "Not now," the voice whispers in your mind's ear, "not just yet…perhaps tomorrow when I am really ready. Besides, I have to…" Excusitis strikes again!

'Excusitis' is a word that was coined by management guru David Schwartz to describe what he called 'the disease of failures'. I think the word perfectly describes the condition that I have seen many of my patients suffering from, and which sometimes appears to creep up on one unsuspectingly. There you are all geared up to start a diet and make the necessary changes in your life, when quietly the doubts start wafting in and out of your thoughts, until suddenly all your good resolve is smothered under a thick blanket of self-doubt, or just plain procrastination.

Try to zero in on the exact reason for the delay in making the commitment and you will find yourself being sucked into a whirlpool of reasons, doubts, excuses, postponements and rationalisations.

Excuse Me!

It's me
It's my genes
It's the food
It's the diet
It's my family
It's life
It's my job
It's my social life
Can't you see…
It's my budget
It's the exercise
It's the time
It's inconvenient
Not now…
Perhaps tomorrow
No, Monday
Or next week
After the celebration
After my holiday
There is no point
It won't make a difference
I can't
Not now, not just yet...

Diet Phobia–Really?

"If it is important to you, you will find a way. If not, you will find an excuse!"

— **Anonymous**

I am not sure such a word exists, but 'dietphobia' would describe an aversion or fear of diets. As mentioned earlier, diets spell gloom and doom, something to avoid at all costs and no matter the compulsions, health advice, or personal realisation and conviction most of us will find a way to put it off or avoid it completely.

This fear or phobia is one of the reasons most diets fail, and it manifests itself in Excusitis—a rash of thinly veiled reasons to put off or avoid the impending necessary changes. The fear of giving up something pleasurable like your favourite foods; the apprehension that one's relationship with food will change forever and food itself will become the enemy; the unpleasantness of focusing or even obsessing over one's weight which one would rather ignore; the very real dread of failure, having tried out various diets in the past; and the reluctance to engage in the many preparations for the diet. These are among the main causes of Excusitis.

The Live Well Diet is based on an understanding of the psychology of legions of dieters who have a strong resistance to, and fear of, dieting, and who routinely fail to maintain a diet after making a commitment to a new way of life. It takes into consideration all the reasons or excuses proffered for not being able to either start or maintain a diet, by creating a varied, flexible, and proactive food and exercise plan, with many solutions for the challenging situations most people face.

Based on thousands of success stories, the Live Well Diet has an answer for every excuse or reason you can come up with, or fear you express, so you can free your mind to take the necessary steps to begin really living well.

Here are some excuses or 'good reasons' why people put off diets, and the Live Well response:

I will begin my diet tomorrow or after that party, holiday, or function. Now is not a good time.

There is no time like the present. If it is worth doing, it is worth doing now. Procrastination is the enemy here, and the chances are if you don't begin today you will never begin at all. There may never be the right time, right place, right mood or right frame of mind when all the stars are aligned.

Take a leap of faith and Just Do It!

Don't wait for the gynaecologist to tell you that you need to lose weight in order to conceive. Don't wait for the diabetologist to tell you to lose weight or risk suffering from diabetes with all its complications. Don't wait for the cardiologist to tell you to lose weight or risk heart disease.

Instead, do what many others have successfully done before you. You can start the Live Well Diet right away—no special foods or gadgets—just the motivation and strong desire to live a better life.

I don't have any will power.

Few of us do. Most of us take the easy way out choosing the path of least resistance. We opt for instant gratification and short-term pleasure rather than long-term good. All that talk of 'living in the moment' sometimes makes us shortsighted about the future.

With this diet you will have enough tasty delicious options and relaxed eating days so your will power won't be challenged as often as you fear.

I won't last out.

This is a common display of a lack of self-confidence. Years of pampering oneself have made one unsure about the ability to stay the course. Here's where you call upon your inner voice that tells you that you need to change your lifestyle. Enlist a family member or friend to provide the emotional support, but remember that external support or monitoring of your progress can only take you so far.

You have to believe in the changes you need to make. If motivation has to come from outside of yourself, let your mirror, scales, and the drop in clothes size do the talking. And remember how much you love and long to hear the phrase, "You have lost weight!" The admiration of friends and family are definitely a bonus.

I hate diet food. Diets are boring.

This is where the Live Well Diet scores over most other diets as there are plenty of delicious options made from ingredients available in local markets and grocery stores. No special diet foods are prescribed—just normal foods combined to encourage a healthy lifestyle. And there is variety—the rotating meal plans provide a range of nutritious tasty dishes that will surprise and delight you. Check out the Two-Week Menu on pages 106-120 and the many options available to you on pages 96-105.

I love food too much—I live to eat!

Then this is the diet for you, as you will learn to both live and eat really well. No more avoiding parties, weddings and celebrations—just suggestions for the event itself, the day before and the morning after. What can be better than that!

I am a part of a family—I can't cook or have meals prepared only for myself. It's too much of a hassle to cook individual portions.

Once again, the Live Well Diet scores over many other diets, as the meals suggested will benefit the entire family. The recipes provided by Master Chef Sanjeev Kapoor are designed to tickle the taste buds of the ardent foodie and serve four persons. Your family will be the unsuspecting beneficiaries of healthy, tasty food and thank you for it. Remember, if you change your cooking methods and food choices to more healthful ones, your entire family will benefit and not just you.

I'm too busy—my lifestyle and work will not permit a diet.

The Live Well Diet is a flexible diet with proactive and corrective solutions for most situations. It has been designed for the modern way of life that involves travel, long hours working away from home, and schedules that can change at a moment's notice. The diet plans can be modified and changed to suit most situations with specific recommendations for foods that are available in restaurants. A list of SOS foods (page 86) that provide a quick burst of energy and quell hunger pangs is another important feature of the diet. With the recommendations for proactive and recovery steps, there is no need to panic or beat yourself up with guilt if you have a momentary lapse—just choose the appropriate solution and get on with it.

I get grouchy and short-tempered when I am on a diet.

Irritability and bad moods while on most diets are usually caused by hunger and a feeling of deprivation. There is no reason why you should be grumpy now as there are plenty of foods you can always have at hand to keep you in good humour. Besides, you will find that it will be impossible to feel hungry, as small meals or snacks in between meals are an important feature of the diet.

If you continue to feel bad-tempered or low despite the meals it may be because you have a feeling of being deprived of the food you have been used to consuming. The trick is to keep your thoughts away from food by distracting yourself with a good film, some exercise, a hobby or a work project that will keep you absorbed and elevate your mood.

My weight and health problems are due to my genes—no diet can fight that!

Genes do play a major role in determining your physical characteristics and your propensity or tendency to suffer from a particular disease such as diabetes or cardiac disease, but so do lifestyle and individual choices. You cannot change your genetic make-up, but you can change the choices you make to counteract the impact of your genes on your health.

I have come across many patients who think they have inherited genetic obesity. However, sometimes it is the family's cooking style that gets passed on from one generation to the next.

A young female patient had lost 19 kg while on the Live Well Diet, but after a year of marriage had put on 15 kg. The reasons she gave me were the cooking and eating habits in her husband's family, the large portions of food served and the large quantities of oil used to prepare the food.

Appropriate eating habits, the right combination of foods and regular exercise will go a long way to combat any negative genetic or cultural influences on your health.

Diets don't work for me.

Most diets will probably not. But unlike most diets, there are so many options with such a high chance of success built into this diet that you will find that it *will* work for you. Of course, despite all its positive result-oriented solutions, you need to give it your best shot and make a sincere effort. There are no miracles promised—the miraculous changes come from a sincere partnership between yourself and your new way of life.

I have a slow metabolism.

The Live Well Diet has built-in metabolism boosters, so before you know it, your sluggish metabolism will be revved up and firing on all cylinders. The diet plans, foods and activities prescribed are designed to activate your metabolism so you burn more energy than you consume. High-protein and high-fibre foods encourage your body to burn more energy, while the large quantities of water and fluids you consume speed up your metabolism, flush out the toxins and hydrate your body.

Diets are expensive. I can't afford to diet.

Your local kiranawala and bhajiwali are the main sources of your food while on this diet. No imported, exotic foods are required, just everyday ingredients. And not the branded, packaged kind either. Your grocery list will include whole grains, pulses, milk, yogurt and plenty of fresh fruit and vegetables. Chicken, fish and eggs will provide non-vegetarian protein, but there are plenty of purely vegetarian options as well. Remember what your mother used to tell you when you wanted to splurge on those burgers or kathi rolls? "There is no better value for money, more delicious, hygienic and nutritious food than home-cooked food!" Delicious recipes provided by Master Chef Sanjeev Kapoor and some from my own collection, will make your mealtimes exciting without resorting to expensive ingredients.

Life's too short. I want to enjoy it to the fullest.

You are right. One should enjoy life and live really well. A change in your diet and lifestyle habits are a proactive way of avoiding a lifetime spent on medication and visits to the doctor because of an avoidable 'lifestyle disease'. Besides, one's life may really be cut too short as many lifestyle diseases are life-threatening.

I am addicted to chocolate—I can't live without it.

Most people love chocolate. But loving something and being addicted to it are two very different things. The question you need to ask yourself when you are pining for your chocolate fix is, "Is it need or greed?" In some cases it may be both, as the only thing that will lift your mood is the smell or taste of the silky smooth temptation. But greed is on another level altogether, and you will need to harness all your will power to control your fixation so you are free of its hold over you.

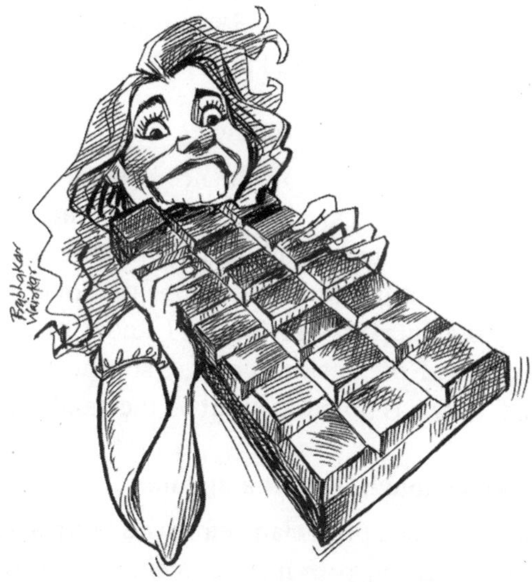

Salads are not for me. I prefer to maintain my macho image and body by eating 'real' food.

Flab does nothing for your manly image either. What you need is muscle not fat. You will find that the Live Well Diet prescribes much more than salads—it specifically recommends foods rich in protein and fibre that encourage the burning of excess fat and building up of muscle in the body. The exercise plans suggested promote the strengthening and stretching of muscles, so not only do you become lean, but fit as well.

I am already eating healthy. I eat only chapattis and dal and an occasional ice cream. I can't understand why I am overweight.

Wishful thinking and selective memory are a common way of avoiding reality or hiding from the truth. Maintain a daily record that will help you keep track of your meals and snacks and reveal the truth about your food habits. You may be surprised to learn how much more you eat between your 2-chapatti meals, and what you eat before and after. A bite of this and a gulp of that can add up to a lot of excess intake which piles on all those extra kilos.

I don't have any support at home.

This is a tough one, for you do need some encouragement and support while you are undertaking any major changes in your life. You will have to call on all your inner resources and strength to make the changes and hope that once the benefits are visible, the support will follow. I know of several cases where because of the positive changes so evident in a person, the entire family has opted to jump on the bandwagon!

I am not well enough to start a diet now.

You should consult a physician before you begin a diet or make any major changes in your life that include increased physical activity. Once you get the green signal, you should have no other reason to avoid embarking on the programme. There is no time like the present and time wasted cannot be recovered.

I am worried about the side effects of diets.

The Live Well Diet is one diet where you will find that there are none of the usual side effects of stringent diets. Far from sagging or dull skin, you will find your face glows with good health. Your eyes will shine brighter and your body will be firmer and more toned up. The food and exercise plans ensure that you lose weight, build muscle and have plenty of energy, which in turn will make you more self-confident and improve your body image. And the compliments will come pouring in.

I am too stressed right now. I have too many family and business problems so I do not have the mental or physical strength to follow a diet programme.

Stress is a very real factor for most people today and it affects your eating habits, as well as your sleep patterns. Emotional eating is one very harmful effect of stress. Many resort to comfort foods to cope including chocolate, foods high in carbohydrates and fat such as French fries, burgers, and rich biryanis. Some even resort to alcohol and chain-smoking to deal with stress.

We all know that alcohol and smoking are addictive, but food can be addictive too, and stress promotes that addiction. So make the time to engage in some relaxing activities like yoga, meditation, and an interesting hobby. You will also find that the food and exercise regime prescribed will have a calming effect on your whole system by reducing the toxins and increasing your metabolic rate, which in turn will lead to a more relaxed you with a more positive outlook on life. And it will show–your new self will attract attention, and perhaps just a little envy!

"I Can't Find My Diet Sheet",
and other Excuses to Stop the Diet, and How to Fight Back!

"People are always blaming their circumstances for what they are. I don't believe in circumstances. The people who get on in this world are the people who get up and look for the circumstances they want, and, if they can't find them, make them."

— George Bernard Shaw

I sometimes find it hard to keep a straight face when confronted with reasons my patients give me when they go off the diet I have prescribed for them. A very earnest middle-aged woman once told me with all sincerity that her husband had forbidden her from 'dieting and all such nonsense' as the food she cooks is not tasty any more. Another bright young lady said she 'forgot' she was on a diet and only remembered the day after overeating at a party. By which time she thought there was no point in continuing with the diet anyway. Another teenaged patient had what he thought was a very good excuse to eat a whole bowl of rocky road ice cream: "I wanted to get the bitter taste of karela out of my mouth." And then, having fallen off the diet wagon decided he might as well eat a few gulab jamuns as well. Stress, PMS, an abhorrence of wasting food, an inability to resist the most fleeting of temptations are all excuses that I have heard for discontinuing a diet plan, and with it, many hours of habit-forming behaviour.

Here are some common excuses for getting off the diet and my responses:

I ate the chocolate pastry because it was in my refrigerator and I just couldn't resist it. Besides, if I didn't eat it, the pastry would get spoiled and I would have to throw it out which is such a waste of money.

Here's a suggestion to begin with: cook the right quantity of food and buy just as much as you will consume, so that you do not end up overeating in an effort to avoid wasting the food. Clubbing several excuses together may appear to strengthen your case for straying from your diet plan (and avoiding waste is always a virtue), but what it is actually doing is weakening your efforts to form the habit of avoiding rich foods.

But, all is not lost and you do not have to give up the whole diet for one slip up. The Live Well Diet has been devised for just these situations when you find it hard to resist a particular food. All you need to do is switch your diet plan the next day so you make a complete recovery and are back on track. What will be a problem is if you keep going on and off your diet plan in yo-yo fashion so you are unable to form good eating habits and begin to put on weight instead.

I attended a family function and I was forced to eat all that rich food as it looks bad and impolite to refuse.

What will look and be really bad is if you continue to be overweight or put your health at risk just to please other people. Stay strong in the face of pressing invitations to fill your plate at a buffet, and make wise food choices. Eat some of the starters like grilled kebabs or steamed wontons; fill up on salads (minus the fat-laden creamy dressing); and stick to the grilled vegetables, seafood or chicken.

The next day switch to a more controlled diet so if you have eaten more than prescribed by your diet, you can adjust your food intake. Better still, plan for such events by ensuring that your diet plan for the day is the appropriate one and that the day before and after you follow the more restricted plan. (See A, B and C Diet Plans page 84).

I have PMS. I am in a bad mood and I am too stressed out. I need something sweet to make me happy again.

This is one time you will be glad you are on this diet as it has just the quick-fix solution you need to brighten your day and soothe your pain. A piece of chikki, a few dates or a square of jaggery will work like magic and lift your spirits almost instantly. Treat yourself to a bowl of soul-soothing soup and curl up in your favourite chair, and all will be right with you and the world in no time. There are many options for those 'poor me' situations—but abandoning the diet is not one of them.

I have been so good for so long, I think it would be okay for me to go on a comfort food, fat and sugar binge for a few days. Besides, I have walked for 15 minutes extra every day and I have earned a treat.

While the diet does have some restrictions, there are enough treats in it to keep your taste buds and cravings satisfied. So there is no reason for you to feel so deprived. If you must, however, do eat a very small quantity of what you are craving—just make sure you don't slide off your plan completely. Look for recipes provided by Master Chef Sanjeev Kapoor that are sure to satisfy your strongest cravings without upsetting your diet plans.

I have been dieting for very long but I have not seen any real results. I am fed up and I just need to go back to eating and living as before. It is just not worth it.

We live in a time of instant gratification and quick results. So it is not surprising that you, too, may want to see changes happen visibly and soon. I cannot emphasise enough the folly of having unrealistic expectations and setting the bar for yourself too high and the goals much beyond your reach. Any change that is meant to be long-lasting and sustained, is one which is slow and steady. It takes time and commitment to reach your goal of good health and a new way of life. Replacing old habits with new ones will not happen overnight. Endurance is key, keeping your eye always on the goal of living well and looking good.

"Excuses are lies wrapped up in reasons."

— Howard Wright

From My Case Files

A woman who had dropped her weight from 92 kg to 58 kg by following the Live Well Diet, brought her husband to my clinic. He weighed 96 kg and confessed he was embarrassed to be photographed with his now slim wife. He felt so bad that he requested his wife to bring him to my clinic. He was so determined to lose weight and look good once again that he diligently followed the diet, making the necessary changes to his lifestyle. It was difficult at first, but he managed to lose 11 kg and is well on the way to achieving his goal of making a pretty picture with his wife again!

Here are some excuses and misconceptions about diets that I often hear in my clinic and which make me smile. Do any of them sound familiar to you?

1. I'll start my healthy lifestyle after the mango season.
2. I remove the oil from cooked vegetables and I eat only the vegetables.
3. I played tennis today. I deserve a vada pav.
4. I have been fasting all day so I can eat a chocolate bar or a plate of bhajias at night.
5. My office drawer is full of chana kurmura, I can eat as much as I want to.
6. Homemade food, even if it is fried, is healthy.
7. I can eat as much healthy carbohydrate as I want to.
8. So what if I am overweight? Nothing will happen to me.
9. What is wrong with drinking tea with sugar as long as I don't drink too many cups a day?
10. There is a wedding in the family.
11. We have guests at home at the moment.
12. My wife packs my tiffin. She doesn't listen to me.
13. My mother-in-law disapproves of diets. She thinks they are just a fad.

As you will have seen, excuses are just escape routes from what is perceived as a difficult or unpleasant situation. You will have to call on your inner strength to stay the course and achieve your goals of living a healthy life with all the benefits it brings.

"Take it one step at a time. It doesn't matter how slow you go as long as you don't stop."

— Anonymous

From My Case Files

This is the story of a young woman who was on the brink of undergoing bariatric surgery when she walked into my clinic, and discovered a more natural, more holistic solution to her obesity.

Her struggles with her weight began when she went to America as a student. Her life there revolved around college, TV and fast food, with almost no physical activity. At the end of four years she found she had gained almost 40 kg, and at the age of 22 weighed 110 kg. Her confident personality became tinged with a sense of inadequacy due to her obesity and poor self-image. When, at the age of 30, doctors told her the only solution to her weight problems was bariatric surgery, she was shocked. She decided to take charge of her eating habits and lifestyle and find a more natural way to lose weight.

She embraced the plans and programmes I prescribed with enthusiasm, determined to strictly follow all my advice. She struggled through the low carbohydrate days, ignoring the headaches and irritability she suffered in the early days of the diet. She soon got used to the smaller portions and found the strength within herself to control her cravings.

Gradually she began to see the results of all her determination and discipline as she saw the kilos dropping off. So completely has she adopted her new food habits that she finds she does not need to refer to the diet plans—she knows exactly what to do in every situation.

Best of all, her self-esteem and self-image have grown more positive and she has begun to feel a sense of pride in the major achievement of turning her whole life around.

5

YOU Have the Power

Food is such a large part of our lives and everywhere we turn we are bombarded by food choices: pictures and recipes on Instagram and Facebook; TV and billboard advertisements; trendy supermarkets, restaurants serving food from all over India and the world; street food carts and overflowing markets. So much so, that food is never far from our thoughts and hard to get away from.

So entwined is food with our lives that we just about finish one meal before we are already planning the next one. Food for many of us has become an addiction and we look to food not only to satisfy our hunger and taste buds, but also our emotional needs. We eat when we are happy, we eat when we are stressed, and we eat when we are depressed. We look to food to soothe our troubled minds, only to find that soon the negative thoughts will surface once again and the cycle will continue.

It sometimes appears that we have surrendered our emotional control to our appetites, and use food as both a salve as well as a weapon. In other words,we may find that we have consciously or unconsciously given food the power to govern our lives.

Therefore, before you launch on a life-changing programme like the Live Well Diet, you need to do a bit of soul searching and ask yourself some fundamental questions about your relationship with food—how conscious you are of its role in your life, and whether you are more emotionally dependent on food than you are aware of.

Ask yourself if you are in tune with your own emotional needs, and do you use food to satisfy those needs? And more importantly, do you love yourself?

It is well known that one's emotional state can have a direct impact on one's appetite and physical wellness. Obesity is often caused by emotional or mental stress, and the link between turbulent emotions and eating disorders has been well established. Poor self-image, lack of confidence, shyness and low self-esteem are symptoms both of impaired emotional health as well as eating and weight problems.

The first step to emotional and physical wellness is to take a long, hard look at yourself and discover all your positive attributes. You will find you have many that you have not really noticed or given too much importance to before. Soon, you will begin to value yourself and believe that you deserve to live a healthy and happy life, free of mental and physical stress. You will also begin to believe that you are worthy of the opportunity to care for yourself and make time to lavish attention on your needs. In short, put yourself and your health first.

One way of staying focused on your goals is to keep a positive image of yourself in your mind. It could be the image of yourself and body as you would like it to be, or as it once was—firm toned body, flat belly, bright eyes, smooth skin, confident, energetic and willing to take on any challenge. Even better, if you have a photograph of yourself in happier, healthier times keep it always where you can see it often and be inspired by the person you could be and indeed, have once been. That self-image will be a like a lighthouse whose beacon of light will guide you to becoming your own best vision of yourself.

As you begin to follow the strategies and food plans recommended you will find, as many have before you, that your confidence in yourself will increase, and your view of the world at large and yourself in particular will become more positive.

A word of caution: do not believe that change happens overnight and that once you have decided to change it will automatically happen. Change can be, and is very often, a slow process that requires a long-term commitment. Which is why crash diets do not work. But make sure that each step you take is a step in the right direction. The smallest changes in your habits and lifestyle can lead to major results in the end. So stick with your resolution to change.

Before you begin the diet you will need to make **a PACT** with yourself to do the best you can for your own health so you can lead your best life.

For that you will need to be:

Positive about the process and the outcome. Put aside any negative fears and doubts and embrace the process wholeheartedly and willingly.

Active physically, and an active participant in the process. Do not wait for things to happen to you. Initiate positive and proactive solutions to every challenging situation you are faced with.

Committed to making the changes necessary to live well. A half-hearted attempt to make lifelong changes only results in turning the clock back, and you will find that you are right back where you started and sometimes way behind.

True to your self. Honesty is the key to success, so be true to yourself and the programme. No lies, no excuses, no cheating on portions. Fooling yourself is a betrayal of who you are and the plans you have for a better you.

And if you think that the diet is your enemy, remember you can be your own worst enemy if you are not committed to changing your way of life, and not motivated enough to take the steps that involve some sacrifice and hardship, even though they will yield positive life-changing results.

And finally, for those of you who look enviously at those pictures of movie stars with their six-pack abs or curvy bodies, luscious hair and glowing skin, remember that that look is the result of commitment, discipline and hard work. No pain, no gain!

Positive thinking, loving yourself, a sense of determination and resolve are more important than all the diet sheets and exercise plans. Focus on the positive results that you will see; the enjoyment of the variety of food choices available to you; the spring in your step after your daily walk or exercise; and you will be enveloped in a glow of achievement and satisfaction at having gained a new life of health and well-being. Celebrate every small step and achievement of inches or grams lost and you will experience joy and hope, which in turn will encourage you to persevere and keep your eye firmly on the long term goal.

Living well does not begin at the dining table or in the gym, but in your head.

As you begin to lose weight, magical things will begin to happen: you will find your view of the world will begin to change; you will find more purpose in everything you do and become more optimistic. The mood changes are directly linked to the hormones that are released in the body when you eat the right foods, engage in exercise and get enough sleep and relaxation.

Your medical reports, which may have given you cause for concern, will slowly become normal, giving you both physical and mental relief. As you see the triglycerides, blood sugar and cholesterol reach normal levels, and the swelling in your limbs, tiredness and breathlessness vanish, you will have much cause to celebrate, which in turn will only spur you on to continue on the chosen path to live well and make it a permanent way of life.

As one patient said to me after losing 70 kg, "Ek admi bahar nikla". In other words, he had shed the weight of a whole extra person that he had been carrying around for so many years.

"It's all in your mind", I tell my patients. You need a strong reason to change your lifestyle and an even greater resolve and determination to make that change happen. The stronger your resolve, the greater the chance of success. It is so easy to give in to temptation, to be hesitant, tentative, uncertain and weak about your decision to change. Your stop-start food patterns lead to yo-yo dieting, swinging from one end of the diet spectrum of not eating at all to the other where you wind up overeating to compensate. Or, you may find you have become a serial dieter who experiments with different diets and harm your body and metabolic processes in the bargain.

Dedication, discipline and determination are the 3 Ds necessary to achieve any goal, and more so when it concerns one's health.

I cannot emphasise enough the importance of a strong will and determination to stay the course. The support of your friends and family are crucial to your success. Connecting with like-minded people who have the same healthy life goals will help keep you focused on your goals.

A positive attitude is also a great asset when making lifestyle changes. I admire those seemingly ageless 'senior' citizens who wear their years with joy and grace, and welcome each day and new experience with excitement and positivity. They inspire all around them with their agile, enquiring minds and supple, energetic bodies. This state of 'ageless being' is evident in the 70-year-old gentleman taking a brisk morning walk; the grandmother who does her own daily shopping and cooking without breaking a sweat; the 75-year-old fitness enthusiast who walks the half-marathon; and the retired school teacher and movie buff who never misses a new film and is the life and soul of every party when she attempts to reproduce one of the dance sequences. Their energy and joie de vivre will put many a teenager to shame, which only proves that age is just a number. It is our mental and physical fitness that determines our state of health. The Live Well Diet has no expiration date—it is a lifestyle that will last forever! So sign up now and gift yourself the power to live a life of health and happiness!

I know I am living well when…

- My skin glows
- My eyes shine more brightly
- My hair is soft and silky
- I can touch my toes
- I can finally see my toes
- I have a distinct waist
- I have lost many inches all over my body
- I can climb stairs without feeling breathless
- My medical reports are normal or near normal
- I sleep well every night and feel rested when I wake
- I can fit into my favourite jeans, kurtas and sari blouses again
- I look years younger than I used to
- I am more self-confident
- I am calmer and more relaxed
- I love being me
- My heart sings as I hear the phrase, "You have lost weight!"

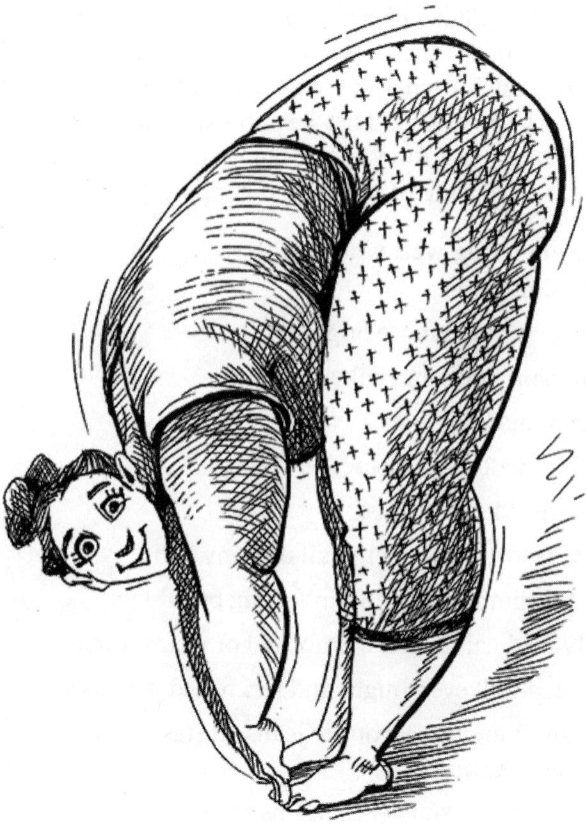

SECTION II

6

It IS as Simple as ABC

Metabolism: Turn up the Heat

Your metabolism is at the heart of any weight loss or healthy living programme. Metabolism is a process whereby food that is consumed is stored and converted within the body into energy to keep your body functioning well. An efficient metabolism ensures that more food is converted to energy than stored in the body.

Any breakdown or slowing of the metabolic process can lead to several diseases, including excess weight and obesity. BMR (Basal Metabolic Rate) is the rate at which the body, while at rest, stores and converts food into energy. The higher your BMR the better your metabolism, and a BMR of over 2800 is considered excellent.

Some factors such as gender and age may have an effect on metabolism. Foods that are rich in protein, complex carbohydrates and fibre, encourage metabolism to function better and keep you satiated longer, thereby keeping your hunger at bay. Physical activity and plenty of sleep also aid the metabolic processes.

As explained in detail in my previous book, *The Live Well Diet*, my diet and wellness programme is based on those foods, plenty of water, activity and a lifestyle that encourage the metabolism to function at its best so that more energy is burned, and only the minimum is stored to help the body function efficiently.

7 GOLDEN RULES TO BOOST YOUR BMR

- Eat foods high in fibre and protein
- Eat regular meals: at least 3 main and 3 to 5 small meals a day
- Drink plenty of water: at least 3–4 litres a day
- Exercise daily: yoga, stretching exercises, walking or functional training
- Sleep at least 7 hours a day
- Relax through meditation and hobbies
- Have body massages: once or twice a week

The Live Well programme keeps your metabolism figuratively on its toes by rotating 3 different protein and fibre-rich diet plans providing different amounts of nutritionally varied foods through the week so your metabolism is encouraged to work at optimum levels at all times.

A list of essential daily foods ensures that you safeguard your basic nutritional needs. Water and nutrient-rich beverages help to nourish the body, flush out the toxins in the system, and improve the functioning of your metabolism.

DAILY ESSENTIAL FOODS

Make sure you include the following foods in your daily diet:

- 3 whole fruits
- 1½ katori (1 bowl) of vegetable soup
- 1½ katori (1 bowl) or plate of salad
- 1½ katori (1 bowl) of cooked vegetables
- 1½ katori (1 bowl) of cooked leafy vegetables
- 1½ katori (1 bowl) of cooked dal, legumes, sprouted beans, chicken or fish
- ½ - 1 katori yogurt

Beverages

- 3-4 litres water
- 2 litres lime water
- 2 cups milk
- 1 glass coconut water
- 3-4 cups green or black tea/black coffee
- 1 glass vegetable juice
- 1 glass buttermilk

Miscellaneous

- 3-4 pieces dried fruit or nuts
- 2-3 teaspoons oil
- Spices and herbs
- Vitamin supplements

The Live Well Food Guide

Based on my experience with many patients, here is a list that I have compiled of foods you should eat and those you should as far as possible avoid. This will help you make the right food choices and act as a ready reference when in doubt. Keep the list handy so you can refer to it when necessary.

Food	Eat/Drink	Occasional, Minimal Consumption
Beverages	Tea, especially green or black tea, skimmed milk shakes, coconut water, vegetable and fruit juices, buttermilk, vegetable soups. Coffee in moderation	Aerated drinks, alcohol, sweetened fruit juices
Bread	2 whole-grain (sorghum/ jowar, pearl millet/bajra, wholewheat/atta) roti or chapatti; or 2 slices multi-grain bread per day	White bread, sweet buns, croissants, naan, sheermal, roomali roti
Dried fruit and nuts	2 pieces of any 2 per day: walnuts, almonds, dates	Cashew nuts, peanuts, raisins
Cereals and grains	Wholewheat, sorghum (jowar), millets (bajra, ragi) flour, quinoa, barley, oats, corn meal and wheat flakes. Rice only twice a week, noodles and pasta: small quantities of eggless whole-wheat occasionally	Refined flour and cornflour. Pizzas, cakes and pastries. Sago (sabudana)

Food	Eat/Drink	Occasional, Minimal Consumption
Chicken	Chicken without skin and fat; chicken salami or sausages	Chicken fat and skin, chicken liver
Eggs	Egg whites	Egg yolks
Fruit	Papaya, pineapple, watermelon, pear, guava, apple, jamun, cherries, strawberries, oranges, mosambi, lemons	Mangoes, chikoos, grapes, bananas, custard apple (sitaphal), coconut.
Legumes and lentils	All legumes and pulses; restrict use of gram flour—mix it with moong dal flour	
Meat		Red meat and pork very occasionally
Milk	Only low-fat or skimmed cow's milk. Total consumption per day–2½ cups including yogurt	Buffalo milk
Milk Products	Skimmed-milk yogurt; buttermilk; yogurt should not exceed 1 katori per day; paneer max 5-6 cubes, twice a week (reduce milk intake accordingly); unsweetened fruit yogurt	Cheese, butter, ghee, cream

Food	Eat/Drink	Occasional, Minimal Consumption
Oil	3 teaspoons per day essential. Preferably olive oil, rice bran oil, safflower oil, canola oil	Margarine, hydrogenated vegetable fat (vanaspati), palm oil, coconut oil, mayonnaise
Root Vegetables	Carrots, turnips (shalgam), kohlrabi (knolkhol)	Yam, suran, potatoes, etc. occasionally
Salt	Maximum 1 teaspoon per day in cooked food	Namkeen, pickles, papads and snacks
Seafood	Fresh fish; eat tinned tuna, mackerel or salmon once a week as per diet plans	Shellfish and prawns
Soya products	Soya flour, chunks, granules, milk, bean curd (tofu)	All soya products must be avoided if suffering from thyroid problems
Spices and aromatics	Unlimited onion, ginger, garlic, herbs and spices	
Sugar/ Sweeteners	Maximum 5 sachets or tablets of sugar substitute per day; eat max 1-inch cube of jaggery per day; eat maximum 1 piece chikki occasionally; eat maximum 2 teaspoons honey per week	Sugar

Food	Eat/Drink	Occasional, Minimal Consumption
Vegetables	All, especially leafy vegetables and salads; mushrooms	
Water	Drink total 3-4 litres of water every day including 2 litres lime water	

Some Important Foods

Almonds: Rich in minerals and Vitamin E, good for the skin, regulates blood pressure and cholesterol.

Amla: Rich in minerals and Vitamin C; anti-oxidant.

Canola oil: Contains healthy Omega-3 fatty acids.

Chicken: Rich in protein.

Dates: Provide energy, aid digestion, rich in potassium, help nervous system.

Egg whites: Rich in protein minus cholesterol or fat.

Fish: Rich in protein and heart-healthy Omega-3 fatty acids.

Flaxseeds: Rich in ALA (alpha-linolenic acid) that improves brain function.

Fruits: Rich in vitamin, minerals and fibre; act as anti-oxidants.

Garlic: Natural antibiotic, blood thinner and lowers cholesterol and blood pressure.

Ginger: Aids digestion, anti-inflammatory and anti-oxidant.

Herbs and spices: Boost immunity and have healing properties.

Legumes and pulses: Rich in protein, vitamins, minerals, fibre; aid digestion.

Oats: Rich in fibre, aid digestion, lower cholesterol, control blood sugar and blood pressure.

Olive oil: High in mono-unsaturated heart-healthy fat; anti-oxidant.

Rice bran oil: High in mono-unsaturated heart-healthy fat, anti-oxidant and rich in Vitamin E.

Skimmed cow's milk: Rich in calcium, whey protein, vitamins B2 and B12; improves the nervous system.

Skimmed milk yogurt: Rich in calcium, protein and B vitamins.

Vegetables: Rich in vitamins, minerals and fibre; anti-oxidants.

Walnuts: Contain healthy Omega-3 fatty acids, anti-oxidants and amino acids necessary for heart health.

Whole grains: Rich in magnesium which helps regulate fat metabolism; aid digestion.

7

The Live Well A, B and C Diet Plans

The Live Well Diet is based on 3 rotating diet plans which are to be followed in a week. Given below is a description of each plan, its advantages and how it is to be used to optimum effect. The diet plans are based on the experience-based belief that restricting oneself to just a few foods is both unrealistic and counterproductive. The 3 different plans are based on the way the body's metabolism functions, aiming to delight with variety and flavour.

THE LIVE WELL DIET PLAN A: The All Foods Plan for a maximum of 2 days

This is the fun plan that, as its name suggests, allows you to indulge in your favourite foods, cater to your cravings and satisfy your taste buds, all in moderation of course. Plan A is ideal for weekends when you can relax your diet, especially if you have to attend social functions, as most people do on weekends. It is also perfect for those weekdays when you have to attend a party, or for when you travel.

THE LIVE WELL DIET PLAN B: The Basic Plan for 3 to 5 days

This is the backbone of the diet and provides the strength and sustenance that will keep you going through the week. A largely vegetarian plan, it provides you with protein, complex carbohydrates and fibre-rich foods on a minimum of 3 days of the week. The large amounts of fibre and protein in the diet will fire up your metabolism and help burn extra calories.

THE LIVE WELL DIET PLAN C: The Control Plan for a maximum of 2 days

A protein-rich and low-carbohydrate diet, it helps your body to burn the excess fat stored in the body. The diet has a detoxifying effect and should ideally follow Plan A, which is richer in nutrients. As far as possible, do not follow Plan C on 2 consecutive days. Plan C is your friend in need—a rescue plan that helps you compensate for any lapses or excesses. It is the make-up plan that will get you back on track towards your goal.

Unlike many popular diets there is a great deal of flexibility in the schedule of the diet plans, so you can begin with any one of the 3 daily plans and proceed with the sequence from then on. You can therefore tailor-make the sequence of your diets to suit your schedule and requirements, as long as you broadly follow the sequence of the plans.

There are no fixed starting points, so you can begin with any diet plan that is convenient, but do try and ensure that Plan A—The All Foods Plan is always followed by Plan C—The Control Plan. You must also ensure that you treat yourself to at least 1 day (maximum of 2 days) in the week to Plan A, so you don't wind up overeating due to cravings or feelings of deprivation!

CAUTION: As far as possible do not reduce the quantity or combinations of foods recommended in the plans. In your enthusiasm to lose more weight, you may decide to skip meals or reduce the amount of foods prescribed. The diet plans have been designed to give you all the essential nutrients in the required amounts. If you reduce them further, you will do yourself more harm than good.

SOS Foods

These are foods that help you cope with cravings or hunger pangs that strike every now and then, provoking you to abandon your diet. Munch on these foods and you will ease your hunger and any feelings of guilt you would have had if you went on a food binge. Make sure you always have these foods at hand in your bag or in your desk drawer at work.

- 2 dates or dried figs
- 1-inch square of chikki made with jaggery and gram (chana) or sesame seeds
- A few gur chana
- 1 kurmura laddoo
- 1 cucumber or 1 tomato
- 1 mosambi, orange, or apple, or 1 bowl of papaya
- 1 square of bitter chocolate
- 2-3 walnut kernels

Eat Just Enough

It is hard to resist generous or second helpings when the food before you looks and tastes so good. The problem becomes even more acute when on a diet, particularly if the food is delicious diet food. You must summon up all your will to stick to the portions recommended by the diet plans as they have been carefully worked out to give you enough nutrition to keep you healthy and your metabolism functioning well.

To make it easier for you, every recipe in Section III (page 143) indicates the suggested diet plans A, B or C as well as the recommended portion size.

Given below is a guide so you can easily measure the desired portions. You can use your regular cups, katoris and spoons to measure the correct amount of food. A set of standard measuring cups and spoons will also be useful.

Equivalents	
Measures	**Volume/Size**
1 tablespoon	15 ml
2 teaspoons	10 ml
1 teaspoon	5 ml
½ teaspoon	2.5 ml
¼ teaspoon	1.25 ml
¼ cup	50 ml
⅓ cup	65 ml
½ cup/1 small katori	100 ml
1 teacup/¾ cup/¾ katori	150 ml
1 cup/1 katori /1 glass	200 ml
1 bowl/1½ katori	300 ml
1 plate	15 cm/6 inches diameter

8

Beyond Food

Losing weight and feeling good requires more than an effective diet plan. To activate your metabolism and shed those kilos and inches you need to exercise and to sleep well.

Get A Move On

An important part of the Live Well Programme is physical activity. A simple regime of a few basic yoga exercises and walking is the best, most efficient and inexpensive form of physical activity. Here are two basic exercise plans to keep you fit and your metabolism working well.

EXERCISE PLAN A

The components are as follows:

- Pranayam: daily, minimum 3–4 times a week.
- Suryanamaskar or stretching exercises: 3–5 times a week.
- Walking: 4–6 km (1 hour 20 minutes) a day (6 days a week).
  OR Yogasana: 50 minutes + Walk 1 hour (6 days a week).
  OR Dance/Aerobics/Floor Exercises: 40 minutes + Walk 50 minutes.
- Whole Body Massage: twice a week.

EXERCISE PLAN B

If you are a regular visitor to a gym and are accustomed to exercise, the following plan will benefit you:

- Pranayam: daily, minimum 3-4 times a week.
- Suryanamaskar or stretching exercises: 3-5 times a week.
- Gym training: Treadmill, Cross Trainer, Stationary Cycle, Elliptical Trainer–60-80 minutes 3-4 days a week.
- Body Massage: twice a week.

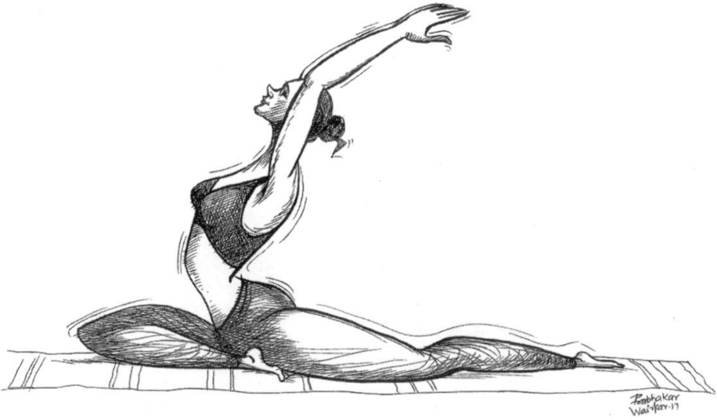

Begin your weight training gradually, starting with basic weights and then gradually moving to moderate, and then advanced weights and functional training. You can do weight training 3 times a week.

IMPORTANT: Please consult your physician and fitness instructor/yoga teacher before beginning any form of exercise.

Just Relax

Numerous studies have shown that stress has an impact on one's health and quality of life. The hormone cortisol is released during times of stress, which is why it is called the 'stress hormone'. Prolonged bouts of stress result in the production and release of excess cortisol that increases appetite and leads to over eating, which in turn leads to weight gain. Stress also affects the entire system and can lead to heart disease, depression, skin conditions such as eczema, obesity, digestive problems, sleep disorders and so on.

Here are some suggestions for activities that will help to counteract the effects of the stress you encounter daily in your life;

- Hobbies
- Music
- Meditation
- Yoga
- Regular body massages
- Volunteering

Some foods are known to reduce stress:

- **Protein-rich foods** such as legumes, chicken, eggs and fish are known to increase the production of the brain chemical serotonin that creates positive feelings of optimism, relaxation, security, comfort and well-being.
- **Warm milk** contains the amino acid tryptophan that is believed to have a calming effect on the system. Drink a glass of milk before you go to bed for a sound sleep.
- **Dark chocolate:** A square will lift your spirits and make you happy.

- **Sugar-free whole grain cereal bars:** Just 1 will give you a burst of energy and fill you with positivity.
- **Dates or figs:** eat 2 to feel on top of the world again.

Mind It!

Your state of mind is crucial to the success of your weight loss and health goals

- Think positive thoughts—try to always look on the bright side
- Deal with those diet-doubts as soon as they surface
- Reduce stress—it causes overeating. Food is the most abused anxiety drug
- Remember that food is addictive
- Control negative impulses with your will power and determination
- Surround yourself with people who have a positive attitude to life

Sleep On It

While you sleep, your body begins to recuperate and regenerate. In a state of rest, your breathing and heart rate slow down, your body temperature is lowered, your muscles relax, and those parts of your brain that control emotions and social interactions are in a state of rest.

Poor sleeping habits, or lack of sleep, cause the stress hormones to increase, and there is evidence that they may also lead to fat accumulation in the body. Sleeplessness affects the production of the hormone leptin that controls appetite and the hormone ghrelin that sends hunger signals to the brain, thus disturbing one's eating patterns.

It is important, therefore, to acquire these habits for a minimum of 7 hours sleep every day:

- Follow a consistent daily sleep routine.
- Exercise at least 5-6 hours before your bedtime.
- Eat your last meal at least 2 hours before you go to bed. Give your system time to digest your meal and your body to relax.
- If you eat foods that interfere with sleep—like those containing caffeine and strong spices—do so at least 3 or 4 hours before going to bed.
- If you feel hungry or restless before going to bed, drink a warm glass of milk, or eat a couple of Marie or digestive biscuits, or a couple of almonds or dried figs.
- Prepare your body for sleep by using relaxation techniques like deep breathing, meditation, taking a warm shower, listening to soothing music, or reading a few pages of a book.
- Turn off the TV, your mobile phone and computer. They need to rest as well!
- Create a relaxing environment: Ensure your bedroom is clutter-free, and your bed linen is clean and wrinkle-free. Spray the room with a pleasant air freshener.

9

Here's the Plan

Your Day on The Live Well Diet

Now that you have an idea about the main principles of the Live Well Diet you will need to plan your daily routine so you can fit all the meals, exercise and relaxation activities into your day. Some will find it easier than others, but it is worth making the effort. The times mentioned are suggestions: you are encouraged to make your own schedule, keeping all the requirements in mind.

Time	Activity	Why
6.30 a.m	On waking, drink 2 glasses of warm water with a squeeze of lime juice	Lime juice aids digestion and has a detoxifying effect on the body
	Drink 1 cup green or black tea	Tea, particularly green tea, is an anti-oxidant which will help prevent or reduce cell damage caused by oxidation
	Drink 1 glass vegetable juice. Eat 1 fruit or a few pieces of dried fruit 30 minutes before exercise	The juice will help further detoxify your digestive system.
7.00 a.m.	Pranayam or breathing exercises, and stretches or surya namaskar	To put you into a relaxed and positive frame of mind and warm up your muscles for further exercise or physical activity

Time	Activity	Why
7.20 a.m.	Walk or visit a gym	To activate your metabolism and burn excess energy stored in your body as fat.
8.30 a.m.	Drink a cup of tea and eat a couple of biscuits or light snack	To help you unwind and relax after physical activity
9.00 a.m.	Eat a nourishing breakfast according to your diet plan	To help you get an energy boost for the rest of the day. Do not skip breakfast.
11.30 a.m.	Eat a fruit or light snack like a few almonds or a date. Drink a glass of coconut water or buttermilk	Keep your metabolism ticking and hydrate your system with nutrient rich foods and beverages.
1.00 p.m.	Lunch according to your diet plan	A fibre and protein-rich meal will provide you with energy
3.00 p.m.	Drink a cup of tea and eat 2 Marie biscuits, or 1 khakra or 1 bowl dry bhel	To prevent the natural afternoon slump.
5.30 p.m.	Have a light snack as prescribed by your diet plan. Drink 1 glass buttermilk	To keep your metabolism active
8.00 p.m.	Dinner according to your diet plan	Eat a light meal that will round off your food and drink intake for the day. Eat preferably 2 hours before retiring for the night.
10.00 p.m.	Sleep for at least 7 hours	Your body needs to relax and recover from the day's activities. Your metabolism will work better if you get enough sleep.

Note: You may exercise either in the morning or evening. You may interchange lunch and dinner menus for the day, only make sure you eat a light dinner at least 2 hours before you go to bed.

Weekly Diet Schedules

Here are some options for weekly diet schedules. Follow the sequence most suited to you. You can change the sequences according to your personal schedules. Just make sure that a far as possible you fit in 2 days of Plan A, 2 days of Plan C and 3 days of Plan B.

Day 1	**Day 2**	**Day 3**	**Day 4**	**Day 5**	**Day 6**	**Day 7**
Plan A	Plan C	Plan B	Plan B	Plan A	Plan C	Plan B
Plan B	Plan A	Plan C	Plan B	Plan B	Plan A	Plan C
Plan B	Plan A	Plan C	Plan B	Plan A	Plan C	Plan B
Plan C	Plan B	Plan A	Plan C	Plan B	Plan B	Plan A
Plan C	Plan A	Plan C	Plan B	Plan B	Plan B	Plan A

Given below are suggestions for each of the three diets which are everyday foods that can easily be prepared in your kitchen. As you will see the options are many, so you have a variety of delicious foods to feast on so you never feel deprived or bored.

Live Well Diet Plan A–The All Foods Plan

Vegetarian and non-vegetarian diet—
maximum 2 days in a week

ON WAKING (Consume all)

- 2 glasses warm water + juice of ¼ lemon
- 1 cup black/green tea + a drop of lemon juice
- 1 glass vegetable juice

PRE-BREAKFAST (Choose 1)

- 1 cup coffee or tea with skimmed milk without sugar. You may use a sugar substitute*
- 1 cup ginger/masala tea with skimmed milk without sugar. You may use a sugar substitute*

Plus (Choose 1)

- 1 cream cracker biscuit
- 2 khakra
- A few pieces of dried fruit or nuts (almonds, walnuts, dates)

BREAKFAST (Choose 1 combination)

- 2 plain or vegetable rawa idli
- 2 medium oil-free dosa
- 1 medium uttapam with 1 bowl sambhar
- 2 oil-free paranthas with 1 katori yogurt
- 1 (2 triangles) wholewheat/multigrain bread vegetable or chicken sandwich
- 2 boiled egg whites/2-egg-white omelette with 2 slices wholewheat/multigrain bread or toast

VEGETARIAN AND NON-VEGETARIAN OPTIONS

LUNCH

- 1 bowl vegetable soup

Plus (Choose 1 combination)

- 1½ six-inch roti + 2 katoris cooked vegetables + 1 katori raita + 1 bowl dal
- 1 katori steamed rice + 1 bowl kadhi or 1 bowl dal + 1 bowl cooked vegetable
- 1 bowl moong khichdi + 1 bowl kadhi + 2 katoris cooked vegetable + 1 or 2 roasted papad (optional)
- 1 bowl veg or chicken fried rice/veg , chicken or fish pulao or biryani
- 1 six-inch thalipeeth + 1 katori yogurt + oil-free lime pickle + 1 six-inch plate salad
- 2 stuffed vegetable parantha + 1½ katoris vegetable raita + 1 bowl chole/rajma/other legume
- 2 six-inch stuffed aloo parantha + 1 katori raita + 1 legume + 1 roasted papad
- 2 medium oil-free uttapam/masala dosa/2 idli + 1 bowl sambhar
- Pav bhaji: 2-3 whole-wheat pav or 1-2 regular pav + 1 bowl bhaji - no butter
- 1½ tandoori roti + 1 bowl dal tadka/1 bowl vegetable curry + 1 plate salad + 1 roasted papad (optional)
- 1 bowl vegetable pulao + 1 katori raita + 1 bowl low-oil vegetable curry + 1 roasted papad (optional)
- 1 bowl vegetable/chicken biryani + 1 katori raita + 1 plate salad + 1 roasted papad
- 1 bowl fada ni khichdi + 1 katori yogurt
- 1 bowl undhiyu + 2 medium roti + 1 katori dal + 1 plate salad

- 5-6 pieces vegetarian/chicken/fish appetisers + 1 roomali roti + 1 bowl dal
- 1 vegetable or chicken Frankie
- Bread omelette made with 4 slices brown bread + 2 egg-white omelette
- 6 pani puri + 1 plate bhel
- 1 plate of 6 dahi puri + 1 plate bhel
- 1 plate dahi vada (4 vadas)
- 1 bowl chole + 1 roti + 1 roasted papad + 1 katori raita
- 6 pieces low-oil kadai paneer/1 bowl paneer dish (6 pieces paneer) + 1 tandoori roti + 1 plate salad
- 1 diet sandwich + 1 glass fresh unsweetened fruit juice
- 6 vegetable/chicken steamed wontons/spring rolls + 1 bowl clear vegetable or chicken soup + 1 bowl noodles with vegetables, chicken or fish + 1 bowl Chinese salad
- 1 bowl Chinese bhel with 1 plate steamed vegetable/ chicken momos
- 1 chicken/vegetable Subway type sandwich without mayonnaise + 1 glass fresh unsweetened fruit juice
- 1 vegetable, chicken or fish burger without cheese + 1 fresh unsweetened fruit juice
- 1 bowl fish or chicken curry (6-8 boneless pieces) without coconut + 1 katori steamed rice + 2 roti + 1 bowl vegetable raita + 1 katori cooked leafy vegetables
- 1 whole or 1 large piece grilled fish (e.g. mackerel, surmai, bekti, rawas) + 1 bowl vegetable + 1 bowl salad or 1 bowl vegetable or chicken soup
- 3-5 pieces grilled chicken + 1 bowl vegetable + 1 bowl salad

MID-AFTERNOON

- 1 cup tea/coffee

Plus

- 1 Snack (see below)

EVENING (Choose 1)

- 1 bowl chana kurmura/bhel puri/moong jor garam
- 1 glass buttermilk
- 2 small diet khakra
- 4-5 steamed wontons/spring rolls
- 2-3 pieces khandvi/dhokla/patra
- 4 oil-free vegetable cutlets
- 1 katori chana gur (1 katori chana + 1 inch jaggery)
- 2-3 pieces corn tikki, corn cutlets or steamed corn

DINNER (Choose 1 combination)

- 3 or 4 katoris/whole fruits (e.g. apples, pears, oranges, sweet lime, guava, papaya)
- 1 bowl vegetable soup + 1 bowl salad
- 1 bowl stir-fried or steamed vegetables
- Note: Keep an hour's interval between fruit, soup and salad

NOTE: Lunch and dinner options may be interchanged

SNACK (Choose any 2 per day)

- 1 glass buttermilk
- 1 glass coconut water
- 1 glass cold coffee with skimmed milk and sugar substitute
- 2 citrus fruits (mosambis/oranges)/2 guavas/ 1 katori strawberries/1 apple/1 pear
- 2-3 pieces of any one: date/almond/walnut

Live Well Diet Plan B—The Basic Plan

Vegetarian diet*—maximum 3 days in a week

ON WAKING (Consume all)

- 2 glasses warm water + juice of ¼ lemon
- 1 cup black/green tea + a drop of lemon juice
- 1 glass vegetable juice

PRE-BREAKFAST (Choose 1)

- 1 cup coffee with skimmed milk without sugar. You may use a sugar substitute*
- 1 cup regular/ginger/masala tea with skimmed milk without sugar. You may use a sugar substitute*

Plus (Choose 1)

- 2 soya/nachni/ragi/jowar/bajra khakra
- 2 oat biscuits

BREAKFAST (Choose 1)

- 1 bowl oats with 1 cup milk
- 1 bowl jowar/bajra/oat upma with chutney
- 1 bajra thalipeeth with yogurt
- 1 bowl bajra/jowar vegetable khichdi
- 2 moong dal cheelas with chutney

***Except for egg whites which are optional, this is a vegetarian diet**

LUNCH (Choose 1 Combination)

- 1 wholegrain flour roti (soya, jowar, nachni, bajra) + 1 katori leafy vegetables+ 1bowl dal or 2 egg-white omelette+ 1 plate salad
- 1 bajra roti+ 1 plate salad + 1 bowl cooked vegetables
- 1 bowl spinach soup + 1 plate salad + 1 bajra roti

MID-AFTERNOON

- 1 cup tea/coffee

Plus

- 1 Snack (page 102)

EVENING (Choose 1)

- 1 glass buttermilk
- 1 katori soya nuggets or 3-4 pieces soya toast
- 2-3 bajra/jowar/nachni biscuits
- 3-4 pieces moong dal dhokla
- 2 medium moong dal cheela or thepla or ragi parantha

DINNER (Choose 1)

- 1 bowl legume salad
- 1 bowl lentils with greens
- 1 bowl veg soup with 2 jowar/bajra/soya/nachni soup sticks
- 1 bowl lightly spiced/boiled or steamed vegetables + 1 jowar roti
- 1 bowl jowar/bajra khichdi
- 1 bowl stir-fried vegetable
- 6 pieces paneer tikki or any vegetable starter with 1 bowl salad

NOTE: Lunch and dinner options may be interchanged.

SNACKS

- 2 pieces soya/bajra/jowar/oat oil and sugar-free snacks (chakli, khakra, biscuits)

Plus (Choose any 2 per day)

- 1 glass buttermilk
- 1 glass coconut water
- 1 glass cold coffee with skimmed milk and sugar substitute
- 2 mosambis/2 oranges/1 pear/1 guava/a few cherries/ a few jamuns/1 bowl dragon fruit
- 2 pieces of any one: date/almond/walnut
- 1 piece chikki or 1 small piece jaggery

Live Well Diet Plan C–The Control Plan

Vegetarian and non-vegetarian diet—
maximum 2 days in a week

ON WAKING (Consume all)

- 2 glasses warm water + juice of ¼ lemon
- 1 cup black/green tea + a drop of lemon juice

PRE-BREAKFAST (Choose 1)

- 1 cup coffee with skimmed milk without sugar. You may use a sugar substitute
- 1 cup regular/ginger/masala tea with skimmed milk without sugar. You may use a sugar substitute

BREAKFAST (Choose 1)

- 1 glass vegetable juice
- 1 fruit/dried fruit milk shake

LUNCH

- 1 bowl vegetable soup

Plus (Choose 1)

- 1 bowl cooked vegetables
- 1 bowl stir-fried vegetables
- 5-6 pieces vegetable or chicken seekh kebabs
- 5-6 mixed vegetable cutlets1 bowl fruit salad
- 5-6 paneer/chicken fish tikkas
- 1 glass strawberry/papaya/apple/dried fruit milkshake
- 1 bowl fruit yogurt
- 1 bowl chicken salad without mayonnaise

MID-AFTERNOON (Choose 1)

- 1 cup tea/coffee
- 1 glass buttermilk/2-3 pieces dried fruit/1 piece steamed corn

Plus

- 1 Snack (page 105)

EVENING (Choose 1)

- 1 or 2 katoris/whole fruit
- 2 moong dal cheelas

MID-EVENING (Choose 1)

- 1 bowl chicken or vegetable salad/1 bowl vegetable soup/chicken soup/4 vegetable cutlets/4 dhoklas

DINNER (Choose 1)

- 1 katori moong or rajma salad + 1 bowl vegetables
- 1 bowl masoor dal/sambhar/rasam + 1 bowl vegetables
- 1 katori chole or matki usal
- 2-egg-white omelette/1 bowl chicken/fish + 1 bowl vegetable or salad
- 2 medium green moong dosa/cheela with mint chutney + 1 bowl vegetable/chicken soup or salad
- 4 pieces Green Moong dal dhokla + 1 bowl chicken/ vegetable soup or salad

SNACKS

- 2 pieces soya/bajra/jowar/oat oil and sugar-free snacks (chakli, khakra, biscuits)

Plus (Choose any 2)

- 1 glass buttermilk
- 1 glass coconut water
- 1 glass cold coffee with skimmed milk and sugar substitute
- 2 mosambis/2 oranges/1 pear/1 guava/a few cherries/a few jamuns/1 bowl of dragon fruit
- 2 pieces of any one: date/almond/walnut
- 1 piece chikki or small piece of jaggery

NOTE: Include chicken or fish only once a day either for lunch or dinner.

IMPORTANT: There may be times you will not feel like eating all that is prescribed. While you may cut down on the quantity, **Do Not Omit The Food Prescribed**, as it contains essential nutrients for your well-being.

10

Two-Week Menu

I have devised a handy two-week menu which includes recipes by Master Chef Sanjeev Kapoor and myself. The menu provides variety, freshness and optimum nutrition and can be repeated after the two weeks are over. Feel free to mix and match the dishes based on the diet plan of the day. With so many options you will keep Excusitis at bay! The two-week menu includes 4 menus for Plan A, 6 menus for Plan B and 4 menus for Plan C based on the Weekly Diet Schedules (page 95).

DIET PLAN A–THE ALL FOODS DIET		
Plan A Menu 1		
7:00 a.m.	**On Waking**	2 glasses warm water + juice of ¼ lemon
	+	1 cup black or green tea with a drop of lemon juice
	+	1 glass **Mixed Vegetable Juice** (page 160)
7.30 a.m.	**Pre-Breakfast**	1 cup sugarless coffee or tea with skimmed milk
	+	2 Marie or digestive biscuits
9.00 a.m.	**Breakfast**	1 bowl cereal [cornflakes, wheatflakes, broken wheat (dalia) or oats] with 2 chopped dates or almonds + 1 cup skimmed milk
	Or	**Scrambled Egg with Mushrooms and Peas** (page 170) + 2 slices whole-wheat or multigrain bread or toast

	+	1 whole fruit (apple, orange, pear)
11.00 a.m.	**Mid-Morning**	1 glass coconut water
1.00 p.m.	**Lunch**	1 bowl **Tomato Basil Shorba** (page 178)
	+	1 tandoori roti
	+	1 bowl **Mushroom Balchão** (page 236) or 1 cup **Handi Murgh** (page 252)
	+	1 bowl **Spinach with Green Peas** (page 229)
	+	1 bowl kachumber
3.00 p.m.	**Mid-Afternoon**	1 cup sugarless coffee or tea with skimmed milk
	+	1 whole fruit (apple, orange, pear)
5.30-6.00 p.m.	**Evening**	1 glass buttermilk
	+	½-1 cup **Kale Chips** (page 209) or 2 small diet khakra
8-9.00 p.m.	**Dinner**	1 bowl **Pepper Rasam** (page 174) + 1 plate mixed vegetable salad
	Or	2 bowls chopped mixed fruit
	+	1 cup green tea
Plan A Menu 2		
7:00 a.m.	**On Waking**	2 glasses warm water + juice of ¼ lemon
	+	1 cup black or green tea with a drop of lemon juice
	+	1 glass **Amla Juice** (page 158)
7.30 a.m.	**Pre-Breakfast**	1 cup sugarless coffee or tea with skimmed milk
	+	1 glucose/cream cracker or Marie biscuit
9.00 a.m.	**Breakfast**	1 bowl **Vegetable and Oatmeal Upma** (page 168)

	Or	**Poached Egg on Vegetables** (page 169) with slice whole-wheat or multigrain bread or toast
11.00 a.m.	**Mid-Morning**	1 glass buttermilk
	+	1 whole fruit (apple, orange, pear)
1.00 p.m.	**Lunch**	1 bowl **Minestrone Soup with Chicken** (page 181) or **Spinach and Baby Corn Soup** (page 180)
	+	1 portion **Five-Spice Fish** (page 246) or **Five-Spice Noodles and Vegetable Stir-Fry** (page 279)
	+	1 bowl **Pomegranate, Cucumber and Tomato Salad** (page 192)
3.00 p.m.	**Mid-Afternoon**	1 cup sugarless coffee or tea with skimmed milk + 1 **Snack** (page 99)
	+	1 whole fruit (apple, orange, pear)
5.30-6.00 p.m.	**Evening**	1 glass coconut water
	+	½ **Spicy Corn on the Cob** (page 208)
8-9.00 p.m.	**Dinner**	1 bowl **Roasted Red Pepper Soup** (page 176)
	+	1 bowl **Moong aur Moth ka Anokha Salad** (page 190)
	+	1 cup green tea
Plan A Menu 3		
7:00 a.m.	**On Waking**	2 glasses warm water + juice of ¼ lemon
	+	1 cup black or green tea with a drop of lemon juice
	+	1 glass **Aloe Vera Juice** (page 158)

7.30 a.m.	**Pre-Breakfast**	1 cup sugarless coffee or tea with skimmed milk
	+	2 diet khakra
9.00 a.m.	**Breakfast**	2-egg-white omelette with 2 slices of toast
	Or	1 bowl **Muesli with Fruit** (page 165)
11.00 a.m.	**Mid-Morning**	1 glass coconut water
1.00 p.m.	**Lunch**	1 bowl **Tofu, Moong Dal and Spinach Soup** (page 177)
	+	1 bowl **Gehun ki Khichdi** (page 267) with 1 bowl kadhi
	Or	1 bowl **Saagwala Murgh** (page 256) with 1 tandoori roti
	+	1 bowl cucumber, onion and tomato kachumber
	+	1 whole fruit (apple, orange, pear)
3.00 p.m.	**Mid-Afternoon**	1 cup sugarless coffee or tea with skimmed milk + 1 **Snack** (page 99)
5.30-6.00 p.m.	**Evening**	1 glass buttermilk
	+	3 **Power Idli** (page 212)
8-9.00 p.m.	**Dinner**	1 bowl **Tomato Basil Shorba** (page 178)
	+	1 katori **Mosambi Salad** (page 191)
	+	1 cup green tea

Plan A Menu 4		
7:00 a.m.	**On Waking**	2 glasses warm water + juice of ¼ lemon
	+	1 cup black or green tea with a drop of lemon juice
	+	1 glass **Mixed Vegetable Juice** (page 160)

7.30 a.m.	**Pre-Breakfast**	1 cup sugarless coffee or tea with skimmed milk
	+	1 glucose or bourbon or cream cracker biscuit
9.00 a.m.	**Breakfast**	Egg bhurji/akuri with 2 egg-whites with 2 slices multigrain or whole-wheat bread/toast
	Or	1½ **Mooli ka Parantha** (page 164)
	+	1 small katori yogurt
11.00 a.m.	**Mid-Morning**	1 glass coconut water
1.00 p.m.	**Lunch**	1 bowl **Murgh Yakhni** (page 184) or clear vegetable soup
	+	2 **Ragi Panki** (page 268) + **Sprouted Hara Chana Amti** (page 286)
	+	1 bowl **Crunchy Celery, Cucumber and Pomegranate Medley** (page 188)
	+	¾ cup (¾ katori) **Chocolate Phirni** (page 302)
3.00 p.m.	**Mid-Afternoon**	1 cup tea or coffee or 1 glass cold coffee + 1 **Snack** (page 99)
5.30-6.00 p.m.	**Evening**	1 portion plain or masala chaas
	+	1 bowl **Kachche Kele ki Pav Bhaji** (page 206)
8-9.00 p.m.	**Dinner**	1 bowl **Oriental Mixed Vegetable Soup** (page 171)
	+	1 whole fruit
	+	1 cup green tea

DIET PLAN B–THE BASIC DIET		
Plan B Menu 1		
7:00 a.m.	**On Waking**	2 glasses warm water + juice of ¼ lemon
	+	1 cup black or green tea + a drop of lemon juice
	+	1 glass carrot juice
7.30 a.m.	**Pre-Breakfast**	1 cup sugarless coffee or tea with skimmed milk
	+	2 methi khakra or 1 **Oatmeal Bar** without custard (page 304)
9.00 a.m.	**Breakfast**	Omelette with 2 egg whites and mushrooms
	Or	2-3 **Kanchipuram Idli** (page 163) with chutney or rasam
11.00 a.m.	**Mid-Morning**	1 glass coconut water
	+	1 whole fruit (apple, orange, pear)
1.00 p.m.	**Lunch**	1 **Soya Parantha** (page 271)
	+	2-3 **Masaledar Karele** (page 233)
	+	1 bowl **Doodhi Chana Dal** (page 290)
	+	1 whole fruit (apple, orange, pear)
3.00 p.m.	**Mid-Afternoon**	1 cup sugarless coffee or tea with skimmed milk + 1 **Snack** (page 102)
5.30-6.00 p.m.	**Evening**	1 glass buttermilk
	+	1 **Corn and Sprouted Bean Burrito** (page 205)
8-9.00 p.m.	**Dinner**	1 bowl **Methi Varan** (page 294)
	+	½ cup (1 small katori) **Apple Basoondi** (page 298)

Plan B Menu 2		
7:00 a.m.	**On Waking**	2 glasses warm water + juice of ¼ lemon
	+	1 cup black or green tea + a drop of lemon juice
	+	1 glass **Wheat Grass Shikanji** (page 157)
7.30 a.m.	**Pre-Breakfast**	1 cup sugarless coffee or tea with skimmed milk
	+	2 soya/nachni/ragi/jowar/bajra khakra or 2 oat cookies
9.00 a.m.	**Breakfast**	1-1½ anda parantha with egg whites
	Or	2 **Set Dosa** (page 166)
	+	1 whole fruit (apple, orange, pear)
11.00 a.m.	**Mid-Morning**	1 glass coconut water
	+	1 whole fruit (apple, orange, pear)
1.00 p.m.	**Lunch**	1 bowl **Jau aur Subziyon ka Shorba** (page 172)
	+	1 bowl **Sing nu Shaak** (page 238)
	+	2 roti
	+	1 whole fruit (apple, orange, pear)
3.00 p.m.	**Mid-Afternoon**	1 cup sugarless coffee or tea with skimmed milk + 1 **Snack** (page 102)
5.30-6.00 p.m.	**Evening**	1 glass buttermilk
	+	3 pieces **Spicy Moong Dal Dhokla** (page 211)
8-9.00 p.m.	**Dinner**	1½ **Bajra Methi na Dhebra** (page 274)
	+	1 bowl cucumber raita
	+	½ cup (1 small katori) **Rawa Kesari** (page 305)

Plan B Menu 3		
7:00 a.m.	**On Waking**	2 glasses warm water + juice of ¼ lemon
	+	1 cup black or green tea + a drop of lemon juice
	+	1 glass **Lauki ka Juice** (page 150)
7.30 a.m.	**Pre-Breakfast**	1 cup sugarless coffee or tea with skimmed milk
	+	2 soya/nachni/ragi/jowar/bajra khakra or 2 **Oatmeal Bars** (page 304) without custard
9.00 a.m.	**Breakfast**	2 poached or boiled egg whites with 2 whole-wheat toasts
	Or	2 **Sooji Pancakes** (page 167)
	+	1 whole fruit (apple, orange)
11.00 a.m.	**Mid-Morning**	1 glass coconut water
	+	1 whole fruit (apple, orange, pear)
1.00 p.m.	**Lunch**	1 bowl **Oriental Mixed Vegetable Soup** (page 171)
	+	1 bowl **Carrot and Onion Florentine** (page 224)
	+	1 bowl **Fruit and Capsicum Kachumber** (page 189)
	+	1 whole fruit (apple, orange, pear)
3.00 p.m.	**Mid-Afternoon**	1 cup sugarless coffee or tea with skimmed milk + 1 **Snack** (page 102)
5.30-6.00 p.m.	**Evening**	1 glass buttermilk
	+	2 **Ragi Idli** (page 210) with sambhar or rasam
8-9.00 p.m.	**Dinner**	2 **Pyaaz aur Pudine ki Roti** (page 272)
	+	1 bowl **Dal Khilma** (page 288)
	+	1 whole fruit (apple, orange, pear)

Plan B Menu 4		
7:00 a.m.	**On Waking**	2 glasses warm water + juice of ¼ lemon
	+	1 cup black or green tea + a drop of lemon juice
	+	1 glass **Peppy Tomato Juic**e (page 153)
7.30 a.m.	**Pre-Breakfast**	1 cup sugarless coffee or tea with skimmed milk
	+	2 soya/nachni/ragi/jowar/bajra khakra or 2 **Oatmeal Bars** (page 304) without custard
9.00 a.m.	**Breakfast**	Masala Omelette with 2 egg whites
	Or	1½ **Buttermilk Pancakes** (page 161)
	+	1 whole fruit (apple, orange, pear)
11.00 a.m.	**Mid-Morning**	1 glass coconut water
	+	1 whole fruit (apple, orange, pear)
1.00 p.m.	**Lunch**	1 bowl **Cauliflower Santa Fé** (page 231)
	+	1 bowl **Apple, Barley and Pumpkin Seed Salad** (page 195)
	+	2 slices whole-wheat or multi grain bread
	+	1 whole fruit (apple, orange, pear)
3.00 p.m.	**Mid-Afternoon**	1 cup sugarless coffee or tea with skimmed milk + 1 **Snack** (page 102)
5.30-6.00 p.m.	**Evening**	1 glass buttermilk
	+	2 **Ragi Dosa** (page 213)
8-9.00 p.m.	**Dinner**	1 bowl mixed vegetable soup
	+	1 bowl **Chickpea and Red Capsicum Salad** (page 187)
	+	¾ cup (¾ katori) **Moong Dal Halwa** (page 303)

Plan B Menu 5		
7:00 a.m.	**On Waking**	2 glasses warm water + juice of ¼ lemon
	+	1 cup black or green tea + a drop of lemon juice
	+	1 glass palak juice
7.30 a.m.	**Pre-Breakfast**	1 cup sugarless coffee or tea with skimmed milk
	+	2 soya/nachni/ragi/jowar/bajra khakra or 2 **Oatmeal Bars** (page 304) without custard
9.00 a.m.	**Breakfast**	Tomato or masala egg-white omelette/bhurji with 2 egg whites
	Or	2 **Doodhi Thepla** (page 162)
	+	1 whole fruit (apple, orange, pear)
11.00 a.m.	**Mid-Morning**	1 glass coconut water
	+	1 whole fruit (apple, orange, pear)
1.00 p.m.	**Lunch**	1 bowl **Dal Mizaaz** (page 284)
	+	1 bowl palak sabzi
	+	1 whole fruit (apple, orange, pear)
3.00 p.m.	**Mid-Afternoon**	1 cup sugarless coffee or tea with skimmed milk + 1 **Snack** (page 102)
5.30-6.00 p.m.	**Evening**	1 glass buttermilk
	+	2 **Soya Shaami Kababs** (page 214)
8-9.00 p.m.	**Dinner**	1 bowl (1½ katori) **Jau aur Subziyon ka Shorba** (page 172)
	+	2 whole-wheat soup sticks
	+	¾ cup (¾ katori) **Moong Dal Halwa** (page 303)

Plan B Menu 6		
7:00 a.m.	**On Waking**	2 glasses warm water + juice of ¼ lemon
	+	1 cup black or green tea + a drop of lemon juice
	+	1 glass **Tangy Cucumber and Celery Juice** (page 154)
7.30 a.m.	**Pre-Breakfast**	1 cup sugarless coffee or tea with skimmed milk
	+	2 soya/nachni/ragi/jowar/bajra khakra or 2 **Oatmeal Bars** (page 304) without custard
9.00 a.m.	**Breakfast**	1 katori oats with dried fruit and skimmed milk
	Or	2 **Scrambled Eggs with Mushrooms and Peas** (page 170)
	+	1 whole fruit (apple, orange, pear)
11.00 a.m.	**Mid-Morning**	1 glass coconut water
	+	1 whole fruit (apple, orange, pear)
1.00 p.m.	**Lunch**	1 bowl **Broccoli in Orange Sauce** (page 237)
	+	1 slice whole-wheat or multi grain bread
	+	1 bowl **Quinoa, Pomegranate and Spinach Salad** (page 196)
	+	1 whole fruit (apple, orange, pear)
3.00 p.m.	**Mid-Afternoon**	1 cup sugarless coffee or tea with skimmed milk + 1 **Snack** (page 102)
5.30-6.00 p.m.	**Evening**	1 glass buttermilk
	+	1 **Vegetable Thepla** (page 270) with chutney
8-9.00 p.m.	**Dinner**	1 bowl **Tofu, Moong Dal and Spinach Soup** (page 177)
	+	2 soya soup sticks
	+	½ cup (1 small katori) **Ginger and Oatmeal Halwa** (page 300)

DIET PLAN C–THE CONTROL DIET		
Plan C Menu 1		
7:00 a.m.	**On Waking**	2 glasses warm water + juice of ¼ lemon
	+	1 cup black or green tea + a drop of lemon juice
7.30 a.m.	**Pre-Breakfast**	1 cup sugarless coffee or tea with skimmed milk
9.00 a.m.	**Breakfast**	1 glass **Amla Juice** (page 158)
	+	1 whole fruit (apple, orange, pear)
11.00 a.m.	**Mid-Morning**	1 glass coconut water
1.00 p.m.	**Lunch**	1 bowl (½ katori) **Pepper Rasam** (page 174) or 1 bowl (½ katori) **Murgh Yakhni** (page 184)
	+	1 bowl (½ katori) **Arbi ki Kadhi** (page 283)
	+	1 bowl (½ katori) **Achaari Baingan** (page 230)
	+	1 whole fruit (apple, orange, pear)
3.00 p.m.	**Mid-Afternoon**	1 cup sugarless coffee or tea with skimmed milk + 1 **Snack** (page 105)
5.30-6.00 p.m.	**Evening**	1 glass buttermilk
8-9.00 p.m.	**Dinner**	2 **Soya Shaami Kababs** (page 214)
	Or	1 portion **Mahi Tikka Lehsuni** (page 216)
	+	1 bowl (½ katori) green salad
	+	1 **Corn and Sprouted Bean Burrito** (page 205)
8-9.00 p.m.	**Dinner**	1 bowl (½ katori) **Methi Varan** (page 294)
	+	½ cup (1 small katori) **Apple Basoondi** (page 298)

Plan C Menu 2		
7:00 a.m.	**On Waking**	2 glasses warm water + juice of ¼ lemon
	+	1 cup black or green tea + a drop of lemon juice
7.30 a.m.	**Pre-Breakfast**	1 cup sugarless coffee or tea with skimmed milk
9.00 a.m.	**Breakfast**	1 glass **Aloe Vera Juice** (page 158)
	+	1 whole fruit (apple, orange, pear)
11.00 a.m.	**Mid-Morning**	1 glass coconut water
1.00 p.m.	**Lunch**	1 bowl (1½ katori) **Tofu, Moong Dal and Spinach Soup** (page 177)
	+	1 bowl (½ katori) **Salade Niçoise** (page 200) or **Sprouted Fenugreek Salad** (page 194)
	+	1 whole fruit (apple, orange, pear)
3.00 p.m.	**Mid-Afternoon**	1 cup sugarless coffee or tea with skimmed milk + 1 **Snack** (page 105)
5.30-6.00 p.m.	**Evening**	1 glass buttermilk
	+	2-3 pieces dried fruit or 1 piece boiled sweet corn
8-9.00 p.m.	**Dinner**	1 bowl (1½ katori) **Murgh Pudina Shorba** (page 185) or 1 bowl (1½ katori) **Spinach Baby Corn Soup** (page 180)
	+	1 cup (medium katori) **Fresh Fruit Yogurt** (page 299)

Plan C Menu 3		
7:00 a.m.	**On Waking**	2 glasses warm water + juice of ¼ lemon
	+	1 cup black or green tea + a drop of lemon juice
7.30 a.m.	**Pre-Breakfast**	1 cup sugarless coffee or tea with skimmed milk
9.00 a.m.	**Breakfast**	1 glass **Peppy Tomato Juice** (page 153)
	+	1 whole fruit (apple, orange, pear)
11.00 a.m.	**Mid-Morning**	1 glass coconut water
1.00 p.m.	**Lunch**	1 bowl (1½ katori) **Hot and Sour Shredded Chicken Soup** (page 186)
	Or	1½ **Ragi aur Tofu Parantha** (page 275) and kachumber
	+	1 whole fruit (apple, orange, pear)
3.00 p.m.	**Mid-Afternoon**	1 cup sugarless coffee or tea with skimmed milk + 1 **Snack** (page 105)
5.30-6.00 p.m.	**Evening**	1 glass buttermilk
	+	2-3 pieces dried fruit or 1 piece boiled sweet corn
8-9.00 p.m.	**Dinner**	1 bowl (1½ katori) **Soya Nuggets with Mushrooms** (page 242) or portion **Grilled Fish with Salsa** (page 248) or 1 portion **Spiced Chicken Bites** (page 264)
	+	1 bowl (1½ katori) **Fruit and Capsicum Kachumber** (page 189)

Plan C Menu 4		
7:00 a.m.	**On Waking**	2 glasses warm water + juice of ¼ lemon
	+	1 cup black or green tea + a drop of lemon juice
7.30 a.m.	**Pre-Breakfast**	1 cup sugarless coffee or tea with skimmed milk
9.00 a.m.	**Breakfast**	1 glass **Mixed Vegetable Juice** (page 160)
	+	1 whole fruit (apple, orange, pear)
11.00 a.m.	**Mid-Morning**	1 glass coconut water
1.00 p.m.	**Lunch**	1 bowl clear vegetable soup
	+	1 bowl (1½ katori) **Soya Keema** (page 239) or **Baked Fish in Red Masala** (page 244) or 1 portion **Greek-Style Yogurt Chicken** (page 250)
	+	1 whole fruit (apple, orange, pear)
3.00 p.m.	**Mid-Afternoon**	1 cup sugarless coffee or tea with skimmed milk +1 **Snack** (page 105)
5.30-6.00 p.m.	**Evening**	1 glass buttermilk
	+	2-3 pieces dried fruit or 1 piece boiled sweet corn
8-9.00 p.m.	**Dinner**	1 bowl (1½ katori) soya chunk masala or 2 pieces 1 portion **Bhapa Ilish** (page 243) or **Chettinaad Grilled Chicken** (page 262)
	+	1 bowl kachumber

From My Case Files

A very worried and overweight 39-year old young man with a heart condition and suffering from Type 2 diabetes came to my clinic for help. I explained to him that Type 2 diabetes is a very common disease which usually affects adults. It is caused by the insufficient production or release of insulin in the body, resulting in a build up of sugar in the blood. Type 2 diabetes is also considered to be a 'lifestyle disease' as it is often caused by stress, poor eating habits and obesity. It can therefore be controlled largely by lifestyle changes and healthy eating habits. He eagerly embraced the Live Well Diet and within a short span of time had lost 9 kgs and found that his blood sugar levels had returned to normal.

He loved to eat. He was what is called a foodie who indulged his appetite for good food at every opportunity. However, his over-the-top eating habits soon caught up with him and at age 37 he weighed 93 kg. and had developed an embarrassing potbelly. He had decided to do something about it, but unfortunately met with an accident which damaged both his knees leaving him unable to walk or exercise. This was a challenging case but with his determination and my guidance, he began to change his eating habits, including eating plenty of leafy vegetables. His weight came down to 82 kg and encouraged by this success he is determined to make the Live Well Diet a way of life. Best of all he is still a foodie!

11

Diet Busters

You try as hard as you can to strictly follow a diet plan but well-meaning people and a host of situations seem to want to sabotage your efforts. Below are some examples of those pesky diet busters with solutions to resist the temptation to give it up 'just this once'. Remember, to form the right habits, you have to persist in the new behaviour until the actions and attitude have become part of yourself. Also, keep your eye on the goal of hearing people remark on how much weight you have lost.

Friends and Family

Yes, loving, well-meaning, supportive friends and family can wind up becoming enemies of your resolve. As good friends, they may, with all the best intentions in the world, tell you that it won't make a difference if you have that ice cream or samosa, 'once in a while'. With a wink and a laugh they urge you to throw caution and better sense to the wind and serve yourself a helping of gulab jamun with a dollop of ice cream just this once!

Be firm, be gentle and spurn all those well-meaning offers with a wink and a laugh of your own! And, if there is too much pressure, use one of the tried and tested 'excuses' some of my patients find useful: "I am dying to eat these yummy kachoris, but I must say no as my acidity is playing up." Or "Sorry, the pizza looks delicious, but I am fasting today."

If you are a parent, another temptation you will have to resist is polishing off the food left by your child on his plate. "To waste food is a sin", you tell yourself as you spoon the leftover ice cream or biryani into your mouth. Again, storing small portions of leftovers is a nuisance, so rather than empty the plate into the garbage bin, you gulp down the remaining food, reassuring yourself that a few spoons extra will not make a difference. But they do, and the habit of eating leftover portions is one that is best broken.

Just make sure only the right amount of food is cooked in your home. If any food remains, give it away (as long as it is fresh) to people in need.

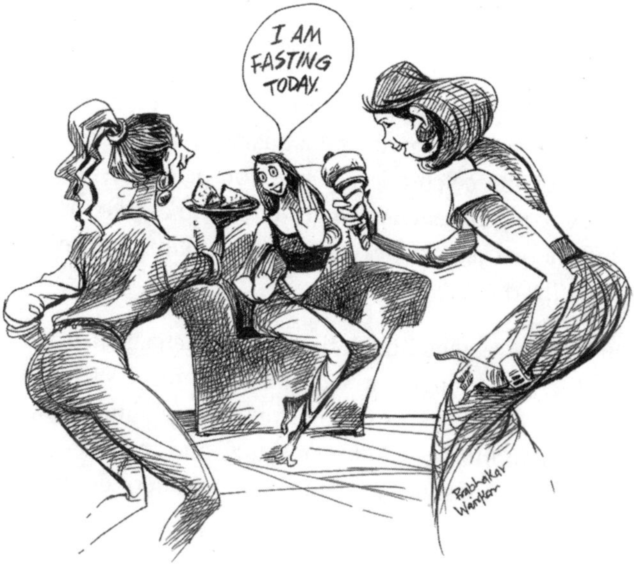

Celebrations

You have to arm yourself against the onslaught of family dinners and celebrations, for that is when everyone is expected to leave diets at the door and participate fully in the hungama. The best strategy is to embark on Plan C (the Control Plan) the day before and repeat it the day after the celebration.

At the event, platters of glistening puris will puff up in expectation, mounds of buttery pulaos will beckon, and rich red curries will shimmer in anticipation as you approach the buffet. As you enter, trays bearing pakoras, kebabs and koftas will waft around you leaving a trail of unctuous aroma in their wake; sugary neon cocktails and creamy lassis will swirl past you in a dance of desire, luring you with their charms.

Taste everything, eat nothing!

It will take all your will power to resist, but resist you must. Give yourself a break by eating a snack or small meal before you leave for the celebration. Once you get there, if you are on Plan A, you can reach for a grilled kebab or two, discreetly wipe off the excess grease with your napkin, and enjoy the barbecued flavours.

Ask for an unsweetened fresh lime soda or chaas, if available, and revel in the strength of will you have displayed. If your tiny purse or your pockets will permit, smuggle in a square of chikki or a handful of walnuts or dates, and munch on them in between the gupshup. Just make sure others don't poach your stash!

As for the buffet, pile your plate high with the salads, (no creamy dressing, please) grilled veggies and fish, chicken, or paneer without the gravy. Give the pulaos and biryanis a miss and opt for roti minus the ghee or butter. Dal is always a good option provided it is not enriched with cream or butter.

Steer clear of the dessert table if you can, but help yourself to fresh fruit (minus the custard or sauce) if it is on offer.

The best advice I can give to you is "taste everything, eat nothing!" That way you will not feel deprived when confronted by a grand buffet. Another trick: eat and drink slowly and hold onto your glass and plate for a longer time than usual, so you are not tempted to refill either.

And finally, remember, the next day Plan C and its deliciously simple fare will be the perfect answer for the day after the night before!

Entertaining at home

Everyone wants to entertain in style and play the perfect host by serving a variety of dishes and keeping the drinks flowing so the guests leave both satisfied and impressed.

You can go one step further and impress your guests with your creative take on 'diet food' by serving up delicious food in interesting ways.

Your dining table could groan with platters filled high with every imaginable delicacy, each one with a nutritious twist that your unsuspecting guests will rave over. Draw liberally from the recipes offered by Master Chef Sanjeev Kapoor and treat your guests to both exotic beverages and lip-smacking food that they will keep coming back for more. If you stick to the basic principles of eating foods rich in fibre and protein with plenty of fresh vegetables and salads, and inventive desserts based on fresh fruit, you can produce delectable food to convince your guests to follow you on the path to living well!

Given below is an entire menu for a party menu including dishes that you will find in this book.

PARTY MENU

(Choose 1 or more dishes for each course)

Drinks

Watermelon and Apple Cooler (page 156)
Citrus Twister (page 148)

Soups

Roasted Red Pepper Soup (page 176)
Murgh Yakhni (page 184)

Salads

Apple Barley and Pumpkin Seed Salad (page 195)
Grilled Chicken and Mushroom Salad (page 202)

Snacks

Kale Chips (page 209)
Soya Shaami Kababs (page 214)
Mahi Tikka Lehsuni (page 216)
Yakitori Chicken with Spring Onions (page 222)

Main Course

Masaledar Tofu Bhurji (page 232)
Broccoli in Orange Sauce (page 237)
Five-Spice Fish (page 246)
Tamatar Murgh Kofta (page 260)

Cereals and Lentils

Mushroom Quinoa Risotto (page 266)
Dal Mizaaz (page 284)

Accompaniment

Pickled Cucumbers (page 297)

Desserts

Chocolate Phirni (page 302)
Quinoa Pistachio Bars (page 306)

Travel

As you prepare for your business trip or holiday, plan ahead for the meals you can enjoy and any supplementary foods you need to take along. Opting for Plan C the day before you travel will make room for any impulsive or unforeseen food challenges. Diet A will be your plan of choice on the days you travel so you will have ample room to manoeuvre around restaurant and hotel menus. Whenever possible, slip in a Plan C or Plan B to balance things out. When you get back home, look forward to the simple life following Plan C and Plan B alternately for a few days.

Fatigue

Fatigue is the foe of the faithful dieter. You are at your weakest and most vulnerable when you feel drained of all energy, and all you want is that one bite or sip of that special something that you know will work like magic, soothing your aching muscles and lifting your flagging spirits. Reach into your pocket or handbag instead and bring out that packet of dried fruit or square of chikki, the piece of fruit, or the tetra pack of chaas and you will find that they too work like magic! And when you can, treat yourself to a body massage or a warm soothing bath that will wash the aches and pains away.

Stress

Stress acts like an appetite stimulant—craving for something sweet and satisfying to increase blood sugar and calm all those turbulent emotions. Inappropriate foods are like drugs that give you a rush of positive vibes and then let you down with a crash. As far as possible, find a way to keep your thoughts away from food and try some non-food stress busters: take a warm bath, do some stretches which will ease those tense muscles, or put on your earphones and listen to some soothing music or positive mantras. Take a walk, and if all else fails, make yourself a steaming cup of green tea, grab a couple of Marie or digestive biscuits and relax in a quiet place until you feel good again.

Moods

A bad mood or feeling low can be a serious diet buster. However, if you are constantly feeling low and depressed, you may need to see a counselor or therapist who will help you identify the reasons for your negative feelings and find solutions to your problems.

It is well known that one of the reasons for a feeling of despondency could be a low level of the chemical serotonin in your body. Serotonin is a neurotransmitter—a chemical that carries signals along and between nerves. It is produced in the gastrointestinal tract and brain, and is believed to affect moods, behaviour, appetite, digestion, memory and sleep. It is also believed that decreased levels of serotonin may lead to depression and feelings of inadequacy or low self-esteem.

It is important, therefore, to ensure that the levels of serotonin in your body are always optimum by eating the right foods and exercising regularly. You may have noticed that you feel very upbeat and positive after a workout or a long brisk walk. This is serotonin in action. Long breaks from exercise will cause the levels to drop and you may once again begin to feel low. Eating high fibre and protein-rich foods are also known to increase the production of serotonin which once again will act as a mood lifter and you will begin to feel good again.

But beware of quick-fix solutions involving sugar or a carbohydrate-rich snack which can leave you more depressed and increase your weight.

Hunger

So often one hears the expression 'I am hungry for chocolate'... or 'hungry for a pizza', or 'hungry for a dosa' or '... an ice cream'. But is that real hunger or just a strong desire to eat what you feel like eating at that moment?

The dictionary defines hunger as 'a feeling of discomfort or weakness caused by lack of food, coupled with the desire to eat'. For many of us, however, what we call hunger may actually be a craving for a particular food at a particular time to soothe a troubled mind, to provide a boost of energy when feeling tired or low, to distract one's thoughts from a difficult situation—in other words as a crutch to help deal with strong emotions. Comfort food is just that—it provides relief and support to tide over an emotionally stressful period.

So how will you know if you are truly hungry, or if a craving is masquerading as hunger leading you to making the wrong food choices?

True hunger appears at regular times in a day and usually four hours after the previous meal. When truly hungry, any food, not a particular one, will satisfy that hunger. A small portion of just 90 grams or a small katori of food, a piece of fruit, or a couple of pieces of dried fruit or chikki will satisfy true hunger.

False hunger, on the other hand, can strike at any time, even within half an hour after eating a meal. Only specific foods will satisfy false hunger, and those foods will usually include sweet or high calorie foods containing plenty of refined carbohydrates and fat.

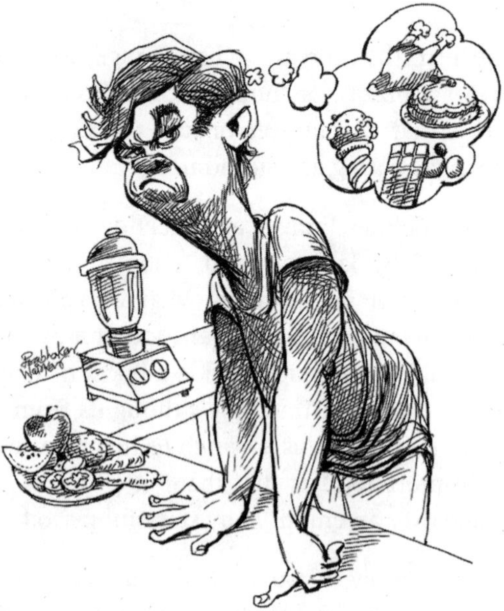

Restaurants

Eating out can be a minefield if you are not well informed about all the good things available to you while on the Live Well Diet. You don't have to order the creamy soup, the fried mutton chops or the rich cheese soufflé. The fragrant clear Thai soup, grilled vegetables or fish with the herby lemon sauce, or the tandoori mushrooms followed by a bowl of fresh fruit will do just as well.

Survey the menu carefully and choose the dishes most suited to your diet. Share portions, avoid the rich side dishes like French fries or buttery mashed potatoes and creamy sauces. Move the bread basket away from you so you do not absent-mindedly reach for a hot roll or naan and order a drink that is sugar-free, light and refreshing to slake your thirst and hydrate your body. You will be surprised how your palate will soon begin to appreciate hitherto undiscovered flavours blanketed under layers of cream, cheese and buttery gravies. Subtle, fresh, herby flavours will begin to grab your attention and you will begin to delight in a whole palette of tastes that you never really did before.

Street food

Sandwich stalls, chaatwallahs, ice cream stands and pav bhaji vendors appear to share a common mission—to sabotage your diet! They seem to be all over the place and it is hard to pass one without gastric juices flooding your belly and your salivary glands going into overdrive. The simplest strategy is to cross the street! If you absolutely must, and your will is cripplingly weak, opt for dry bhel (sukha bhel) with green chutney, or ragda without the pattice, bhaji without the pav and butter (if you can get the thelawalla to hear your request above the din) and then go home and skip dinner—just help yourself to some clear vegetable soup.

Malls

There is plenty of choice for the live well dieter at the food courts in most malls: opt for idli, burgers minus the buns, roti rolls, steamed corn without the butter, popcorn—no caramel and butter please, kebabs and clear soups. Fruit chaat is an option and salads minus the creamy dressing or salad cream are good choices. Of course, it depends on what your diet plan is for the day. Keep your visits to malls to Plan A days so you can be more relaxed about your food choices.

Supermarkets

You start out with a list of healthy, nutritious, metabolism-revving foods but the shelves laden with bright, alluring boxes and bottles can be hard to ignore. "Pick me!" "Buy me!" they scream as you wheel your trolley hurriedly past. If you let temptation and curiosity get the better of you, you are one step closer to falling. If you begin to fool yourself that Choti would love these chocolate cream treats and Dadu loves the sohan papdi, you are a hair's breadth away from the slippery slope. You will need all your resolve to steer pass those temptations, or steel yourself to resist opening the packet or box when you are in the car on your way home!

The solution: stick to the list! Better still, phone in your orders and if you have to visit the supermarket, make sure it is not on an empty stomach—swill down some soup or chomp on a piece of fruit before you go forth with your list firmly in hand.

Workouts

Yes, even a good work out can put your diet and eating plans in jeopardy. There are two situations to guard against. Firstly, a feeling of achievement after strenuous activity, when you feel you can eat as much as you like as you have been diligent, and therefore have earned a reward for your effort. Secondly, a belief that because you have been so good, you can 'cheat' a bit by indulging in a 'forbidden' food.

Sometimes, you may be tempted to eat more than you should, promising yourself a longer workout the next day to make up for it. This sort of thinking is understandable once in a while, but it can very easily become a habit and soon you will find that you are slipping back into your old unwise eating habits.

Keep a bottle of fresh fruit juice or coconut water to hydrate yourself after you exercise, and a piece of fruit to replenish some of the energy you have burned.

Finally, there is You!

You may have noticed that the diet buster that is common to all the above is you! All the temptations and coercing in the world will not work unless you give in or give up. You are in charge and can make the right choices—you just need to be motivated, prepared and smart.

12

Frequently Asked Questions

I see a wide variety of patients of all ages and from different cultural backgrounds. All of them are concerned about their weight and sincerely want to live a healthy life. There are some questions that I am asked more frequently than others. Some of these questions I have covered in my first book *The Live Well Diet*. Here are some others:

Will I put on weight again after losing so much weight?

If you follow all the principles and recommendations of the Live Well Diet including the A, B and C Diet plans, and follow a consistent exercise regime, there is no reason you should put on weight again. Your diet and exercise should become a matter of routine and habit so you will automatically follow them, and keep you in good health and your weight under control.

I have been smoking for many years. Can I continue to smoke while on the Live Well Diet?

NO! You will have to give up smoking completely and immediately.

I have pain in my legs. How will I be able to exercise and lose weight?

I have many patients suffering from arthritis, rheumatism and back pain who have a problem doing exercises. My advice to them is to try pranayam yoga, body stretches and leisurely walks. Stick to a low-carbohydrate diet and follow the diet plans prescribed. Walking in a swimming pool is a good way to exercise. Do consult your physician before you engage in any form of exercise.

I suffer from headaches. Will they get worse while I am on a diet?

I have seen many patients who come to me with migraines and other kinds of headache, but after some time on the diet, the headaches disappear. My advice is to drink plenty of water and eat small portions with a gap of 2 to 3 hours.

Will my skin become loose and flabby after I lose weight?

Do not worry. The Live Well Diet includes exercise, stretching, fitness training and passive exercise (massage). The process of weight loss is slow, so if your exercise and diet go hand in hand, your body will become firmer and well toned.

How do I know what my ideal weight is?

Please refer to the weight chart on (page 312). Your target weight (+) or (-) 2 kg is ideal for you. If your weight drops drastically below the target weight you need to consult your physician as it may be due to various health factors. If it increases 5 kg above the target weight, you will need to engage in a diet and exercise plan to reduce the excess weight.

If I have a food craving at night or during menstruation, what should I do?

If you have followed a routine of regular exercise and a relaxing activity such as reading or listening to music before you go to bed, you should be able to sleep soundly without feeling any late night hunger pangs. But if necessary, make yourself a dried fruit milkshake or eat a handful of chana gur. The same goes for those cravings during your monthly periods.

I can control my hunger throughout the day, but by evening I feel really hungry. I am then tempted to snack on whatever is around including fried and starchy foods. How do I cope?

If you are following the Live Well Diet you should not feel hungry as there is plenty of opportunity to fill you up right through the day. However, should hunger pangs strike, eat some chana gur, a piece of chikki or drink a dried fruit milkshake. You can also drink coconut water or buttermilk, or eat some natural unsweetened fruit yogurt.

Special Cases

People of all walks of life and of all ages have tried and been successful on the Live Well Diet. The one thing they have had in common is an overwhelming desire to live a healthy life and the determination to achieve their goals. Here are some examples of the advice I give my patients in various careers or stages of life that I would like to share with you.

Pregnant Women

The beaming smile, glow on the face and gentle bump says it all—a baby is on the way! Pregnancy is a time for celebration and delightful anticipation of one of the miracles of life. It is also a time when the expectant mother blossoms and blooms, sometimes, unfortunately, rather too much. The tendency to pamper oneself and be pampered, leads to an increase of weight beyond the recommended parameters—usually about 12 to 15 kg for a woman of normal weight. The more the weight gain, the harder it will be to shed the excess kilos after delivery. So I advise my pregnant patients to eat just a little more nutritious food than they usually do to nourish the life they are carrying. I also advise them to consult their obstetrician before starting the diet.

With the attendant normal hormonal and physical changes during pregnancy and its aftermath, symptoms like water retention, hair loss, sleeplessness and fatigue are common. To overcome the symptoms and get back to a normal rhythm of life, I advise them to make sure they can draw on the support of family and friends to help prepare nutritious meals, make enough time to do some physical activity such as yoga and walking, some meditation or stress-relieving activities together with body massages and power naps. Having followed the diet and exercise plans their minds and bodies became fit and refreshed to enjoy their new role as a mother.

A Female Pilot

One of the interesting cases I came across is that of a pilot who was a woman. This is an unusual choice of profession for a woman, but one that is becoming more common these days when gender is less of an issue in hitherto male-dominated careers. The challenges with respect to lifestyle, however, remain the same—irregular and stressful working hours, frequent changes of locations and climates, travel across time zones for international travel, and high altitude flying which takes its toll on one's health and fitness if not managed well.

To combat all the challenges, I recommended the Live Well Diet with its emphasis on low-fat, high-fibre and high-protein foods and regular exercise and relaxation regime. Keeping the body well hydrated while flying is also very important. As the food provided on an airline is not always well balanced, I suggested she should carry a home-cooked meal in keeping with her diet plan while on duty which worked well with excellent results.

Today, hotel chefs are more enlightened about healthy food and many hotels provide more healthy options on their menus. Wherever she goes, she requests the chef to cook a high-fibre, high-protein meal for her.

A Marathon Runner

Marathon runners burn an enormous amount of energy during their rigorous training and performing schedules. Eating the right foods that will provide them with the necessary energy and build muscle and stamina is naturally of prime importance. The tendency during a run is to cool down and give oneself a burst of energy with a packaged sugary beverage. This may not always be the right solution.

I therefore recommended natural juices and protein-rich dried fruit shakes, coconut water and fresh lime juice which will provide the energy without the negative side effects.

In addition, a high-protein diet to build muscle strength, and a soothing stress-relieving activity to help the body relax and recover after a strenuous run.

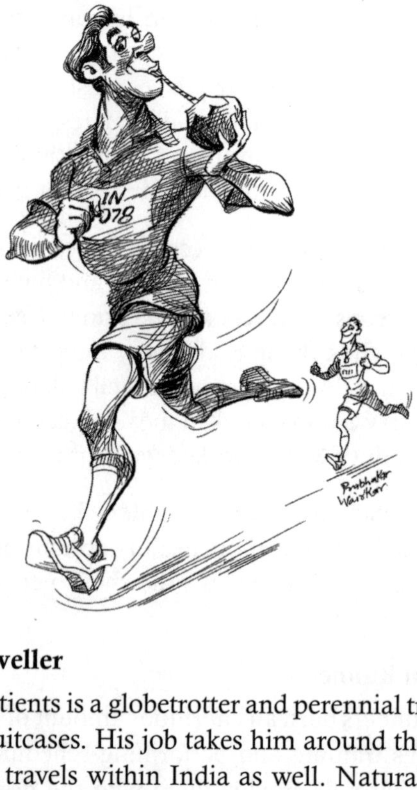

An Avid Traveller

One of my patients is a globetrotter and perennial traveller who lives out of suitcases. His job takes him around the world and he frequently travels within India as well. Naturally, his food habits are constantly varied to suit his schedules and the places he visits. Not surprisingly, obesity and stress were his major complaints. It is a challenge to follow a regular programme that involves specific foods and a prescribed exercise routine.

However, as I explained, because of its inbuilt flexibility, he could follow the Live Well Diet and still combat the problems of obesity and stress. The programme does involve discipline, a strong will power and motivation to live a healthy life and at the same time be able to enjoy the thrill (and necessity) of being constantly on the go. The trick, I told him, is to pick yourself up every time you fall off the programme, take immediate remedial action by choosing the right diet plan (Plan C) including a low-fat diet with plenty of fruit and vegetables and hearty soups to provide energy without the empty calories. Drinking plenty of water is essential while travelling, as is making the time to get in some physical activity—a long brisk walk is best and does not require any special equipment. For those hunger pangs, I recommended he keep some dried fruit or chikki close at hand to stave off the temptation to grab an unhealthy snack. For a non-vegetarian option, I recommended an egg-white omelette which is a good way to keep hunger at bay.

Obese Children

A roly-poly toddler with pink, chubby cheeks waddling on fat little legs is a delight to behold. The photograph of such a child will draw 'oohs' and 'aahs' and be shared on Twitter and Facebook as the epitome of a healthy, happy child. A few years on and that same chubby little child may not look or be that healthy, especially if the fat has continued to pile on. A fat or obese child is not a well child, emotionally or physically. In our desire to provide the best of everything for our children we sometimes make the mistake of overfeeding them and indulging their every fancy no matter how nutritionally misguided. We ply them with chocolates and pizza and unlimited soft drinks all in the name of 'love', creating in the child a dependence on food and an insatiable appetite for rich, often junk, food.

I have had several obese children brought to my clinic. This is what I tell their parents: "As a responsible parent, the health of your child must be paramount." I advise parents to start by leading by example and providing only those foods that are necessary for healthy growth.

- Stop or severely curtail the junk food and packaged snacks that are such a fad these days.
- Introduce a variety of foods, especially green vegetables, to your child at an early age so the palate is exposed to different textures and flavours.
- Introduce healthy methods of cooking such as steaming and roasting as alternatives to fried foods.
- Whole grain breads and cereals, lentils and pulses, fresh fruit and vegetables, milk and milk products, with protein in the form of fish or chicken, should make up the bulk of a growing child's diet.
- Find innovative ways to include plenty of essential vegetables in the diet. Add them to rice, lentils, sauces and soups. Use vegetables as fillings in wraps and rolls. Include them in popular foods like fried rice, biryani, pulaos and pasta.
- Always have fresh juices and chaas at hand so they do not have to turn to soft drinks or packaged juices to quench their thirst.
- A child's education at home should include an appreciation of different foods, regular eating habits and ways to make wise food choices.
- Involve your children in planning menus and preparing food so they understand how to balance a meal to include foods from different food groups.
- Above all, make sure your child gets plenty of exercise and a good night's sleep. Hobbies and learning a craft helps keep the mind and body active, which is also important for the all-round well-being and development of your child.

Be the Change You Want to See!

Write your own success story and measure your gains by the lifestyle and food habits you have managed to change.

Before the Live Well Diet	After the Live Well Diet
Lifestyle	
Sedentary (couch potato)	Active
High stress	Proper work-life balance and stress management techniques
Irregular sleep patterns	Regular sleep pattern (early to bed, early to rise)
Excessive alcohol and/or smoking	Limited alcohol and no smoking
Less intake of water	Proper intake of water
Food Choices	
Red meat	Chicken, fish and legumes
Sugar	Minimal or no sugar or sugar substitute
Vanaspati, butter or margarine	Homemade cow's ghee in moderation
Oily food	Oil only for tadka, and to grease
Deep-frying	Pan-frying, air-frying, baking, steaming, grilling
Bread	Whole-wheat or multigrain bread or roti chapatti
Excess salt	Minimum salt only for taste
Rice	Oats, quinoa, brown rice, whole grains
Refined flour (maida)	Wheat flour or multigrain flour
Gram flour (besan)	Mung dal flour
Coconut oil, sesame (til) oil	Mustard, olive, rice bran oil
Sugary fruits like mango and banana	Guava, pear, apple, citrus fruits
Packaged foods	Fresh home-made food

Finally It's All in the Mind

The difficulty is not getting your body in shape. It is getting your mind in shape!

I have given you the tools, plans, knowledge and experience that I have shared with thousands of patients who have benefited from the Live Well Diet and way of life. It is now up to you to take that first step that will set you firmly on the path to a life of mental and physical well-being. That first step begins in your mind, and it is your mind that will guide your actions and shape your habits. A positive approach, a strong resolve and commitment, and the firm belief that you can and will achieve your goal will arm you with the emotional strength you need to see you through the periods of doubt, low self-esteem and frustration.

You are further armed with lip-smacking, nutritious recipes from my own collection and from Master Chef Sanjeev Kapoor, which will make living well a delicious, healthy journey you can share with family and friends.

So, no more excuses, take that first step and DO IT NOW!

NO MORE EXCUSES
No more: If only...
No more: But...
No more: It's not my fault
No more: I can't
No more: Nothing will happen to me
No more: Just this once...
No more: Tomorrow...
No more: I am too tired
No more: It's too difficult
No more: Nothing will work

"The beginning is always NOW."

— Roy T. Bennett

SECTION III

Recipes

Introduction

One of the fears of going on a diet is that you will have to eat bland or tasteless food. I am here to assure you that that is far from the truth. Guided by this book you will discover that there are plenty of very tasty options for your every meal. The Live Well Diet encourages you to eat the right foods at the right time and in the right quantity so you need never experience a lack of really delicious, satisfying food.

Most of the recipes call for everyday ingredients available at your local grocer, supermarket or vegetable vendor. Follow the recipes and add your own twist to them keeping in mind the foods that will benefit and those that will derail your diet. You will also find recipes in this section to serve to guests at parties and celebrations. A sample menu (page 126) will give you an idea of the variety of dishes that one would never associate with 'diet food'.

You will also be happy to know that each recipe serves four persons, so your family can enjoy the delicious dishes too. In addition, we have specified the appropriate diet plan for each recipe as well as the portion size. Our aim is to make it as easy as possible for you to succeed in making the necessary changes in your eating habits so you can live a life of good health and wellness.

Happy Cooking and Live Well!

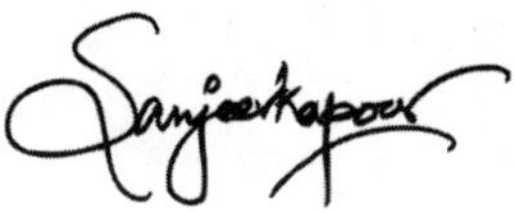

You are a Smart Cookie if...

- You don't peel the skins of fruit like apples and pears, and vegetables like cucumbers and tender gourds. They add fibre to your diet.
- You add plenty of herbs and spices while cooking so you will hardly notice the absence of oil or fat in your food.
- You spray the pan with oil instead of pouring it in to shallow-fry foods.
- You replace the fat in baked goods with apple purée or yogurt.
- To thicken soups and gravies, you purée cooked vegetables, (especially bottle gourd and cauliflower), or lentils.
- You replace mashed potato with boiled and mashed cauliflower as a side dish, or in cutlets and kebabs.
- For seasoning (tadka) you use a small non-stick pan. You add just a drop of oil and stir the spices until they are coated with the oil and begin to roast and change colour.
- To sauté onions (bhunao) you grate or purée the onions, ginger and garlic and cook them without any oil in a non-stick pan until almost dry. Finally, you add a teaspoon of oil and brown the paste to remove the raw smell. Continue cooking as required.
- You remove the skin and excess fat from chicken.
- You regularly use cooking methods that require little oil and preserve the nutrients in the food such as steaming, poaching, grilling, stir-frying and microwave cooking.

Adrak Navratan

INGREDIENTS

75 grams fresh tender ginger, peeled and cut into fine strips

10-12 (60 grams) dried dates (chuhare), stoned and cut into fine strips

½ cup raisins (kishmish)

5-6 green chillies, cut in half

½ cup lemon juice

A pinch of salt

½ teaspoon black salt

METHOD

- Combine the ginger, dates, raisins, chillies, lemon juice, salt, black salt and one cup of water in a bowl and mix well.
- Transfer the mixture into a shaker or a wide-mouthed glass jar with a lid.
- Shake well and set aside for seven days, or until the juice turns pink.
- For each serving, place one tablespoon juice along with one tablespoon ginger and date strips into a glass.
- Add one cup of chilled water, stir lightly and serve.

Diet Plans: A B C
Portion: 1 glass

Citrus Twister

INGREDIENTS

2 cups fresh orange juice

½ cup fresh pink grapefruit juice

4 teaspoons lemon juice

Crushed ice, as required

2 cups chilled club soda

4 lemon twists, to decorate

METHOD

- Pour orange juice, grapefruit juice and lemon juice into a shaker and shake well for half a minute.
- Strain into four glasses and add crushed ice. Top up with club soda and stir lightly.
- Decorate with a lemon twist and serve immediately.

Diet Plans: A B C
Portion: 1 glass

Iced Cajun Coffee

INGREDIENTS

2 tablespoons instant coffee powder

2 cups cold skimmed milk

2 teaspoons vanilla essence

Crushed ice, as required

2 small pinches cinnamon powder

METHOD

- Blend together instant coffee powder, milk and vanilla essence in a blender.
- Pour over crushed ice in four glasses. Sprinkle cinnamon powder over the top and serve immediately.

Diet Plans: A B C

Portion: 1 glass

Lauki ka Juice

INGREDIENTS

2 medium bottle gourds (lauki), peeled, seeded and chopped

4 Indian gooseberries (amla), sliced

2 inches ginger, chopped

15-20 fresh mint leaves

Salt to taste

Black salt to taste

1 tablespoon cumin seeds

2-3 tablespoons lemon juice

Ice cubes, as required

METHOD

- Place the bottle gourd, gooseberries, ginger, mint leaves, salt, black salt and cumin seeds in a blender.
- Add one cup of water and blend the mixture until smooth.
- Add another cup of water, lemon juice and ice cubes and blend again.
- Strain into individual glasses and serve chilled.

Diet Plans: A B C
Portion: 1 glass

Melon Medley

INGREDIENTS

2 cups seeded musk melon chunks, chilled

2 cups seeded watermelon chunks, chilled

¾ cup fresh pineapple juice, chilled

4 fresh pineapple slices

METHOD

- Blend together musk melon, watermelon and pineapple juice in a blender at high speed until smooth.
- Pour into individual glasses.
- Fix a slice of pineapple on the rim of each glass and serve immediately.

Diet Plans: A B C

Portion: 1 glass

Mint Mojito

INGREDIENTS

10-12 fresh mint leaves

4 fresh mint sprigs

4 lemons

1 green chilli

Sea salt to taste

Black salt to taste

2 teaspoons powdered sugar or sugar substitute to taste

Ice cubes, as required

Chilled water, as required

METHOD

- Quarter three lemons and cut the remaining one in half.
- Squeeze the juice from the lemon halves into a stainless steel jug. Put the lemon quarters in it.
- Add green chilli, sea salt, black salt, mint leaves and crush with a pestle or the handle of a wooden spoon.
- Add powdered sugar, half a cup of water and mix. Add ice cubes and shake to mix well.
- Place a mint sprig in a serving glass; add ice cubes and strain the mixture through a strainer into the glass.
- Top it up with chilled water and mix.
- Serve immediately.

Diet Plans: A B C
Portion: 1 glass

Peppy Tomato Juice

INGREDIENTS

7 ripe red tomatoes, chopped

2 inches celery stalk, chopped

Salt to taste

1½ teaspoons sugar or equivalent sugar substitute (optional)

Crushed ice, as required

1½ teaspoons crushed black peppercorns

METHOD

- Combine the tomatoes and celery. Sprinkle salt and sugar, and place in the refrigerator for twenty minutes.
- Process in a blender along with one and a half cups of water until smooth.
- Press the mixture through a strainer and pour into four glasses.
- Top up with crushed ice and sprinkle with crushed peppercorns and serve.

Diet Plans: A B C
Portion: 1 glass

Tangy Cucumber and Celery Juice

INGREDIENTS

2 medium cucumbers, peeled and roughly chopped

2 inches celery stalk, roughly chopped

2 tablespoons lemon juice

1 teaspoon sugar or equivalent sugar substitute (optional)

Salt to taste

Ice cubes, as required

For garnishing

A few sprigs of fresh mint leaves

4 three-inch celery stalks

METHOD

- Place cucumber, celery, lemon juice, sugar and salt with four cups of water and ice cubes in a blender and process until well blended.
- Pour the juice into glasses and serve immediately, garnished with a sprig of mint and a celery stalk.

Diet Plans: A B C
Portion: 1 glass

Tulsi ki Chai

INGREDIENTS

12-16 fresh basil (tulsi) leaves

4 teaspoons tea leaves

1 inch ginger, peeled and crushed

3 teaspoons honey

3-4 black peppercorns

METHOD

- Place basil leaves and four and a half cups of water in a deep non-stick pan and bring to a boil.
- Reduce heat and simmer for five minutes.
- Add tea leaves, ginger, honey and peppercorns and bring back to a boil.
- Remove from heat, cover and let the tea infuse for about five minutes.
- Strain into tea cups and serve.

Diet Plans: A B C
Portion: 1 tea cup

Watermelon and Apple Cooler

INGREDIENTS

½ medium watermelon, seeded and cut into cubes

1 medium apple, peeled and grated

2 teaspoons powdered sugar or equivalent sugar substitute (optional)

Rock salt to taste

1 teaspoon roasted cumin seeds, coarsely crushed

1 tablespoon fresh mint leaves, chopped + a few sprigs to garnish

Crushed ice, as required

METHOD

- Combine the watermelon, powdered sugar and rock salt in a blender jar and blend until smooth.
- Transfer to a jug, add crushed cumin, chopped mint and ice and stir to mix well.
- Add the grated apple and stir to mix.
- Pour into individual glasses and serve, garnished with mint sprigs.

Diet Plans: A B C

Portion: 1 glass

Wheat Grass Shikanji

INGREDIENTS

4 bunches (400 grams) wheat grass

6 teaspoons sugar or equivalent sugar substitute

1 teaspoon black salt

1 teaspoon crushed black peppercorns

Juice of 4 lemons

Salt to taste

Ice cubes, as required

For garnishing

4 lemon slices

A few fresh mint leaves

METHOD

- Grind together wheat grass, sugar, black salt, peppercorns, lemon juice, salt, ice cubes and one glass of water into a fine paste.
- Strain the mixture into a bowl and stir in three glasses of water.
- Pour into four glasses, garnish with lemon slices and mint leaves and serve chilled.

Diet Plans: A B C

Portion: 1 glass

Aloe Vera Juice

INGREDIENTS

2 cups aloe vera juice

A handful of fresh basil leaves (tulsi)

1 inch ginger, chopped

METHOD

- Blend together the aloe vera juice, basil leaves and ginger with two cups of water. Strain and serve.

Recipe courtesy Dr Sarita Davare

Diet Plans: A B C
Portion: 1 glass

Amla Juice

INGREDIENTS

8 Indian gooseberries (amla), seeded

2 inches ginger

2 teaspoons cumin seeds

METHOD

- Blend together the gooseberries, ginger and cumin seeds with five cups of water.
- Strain and serve.

Recipe courtesy Dr Sarita Davare

Diet Plans: A B C
Portion: 1 glass

Pani Puri Pani

INGREDIENTS

4 cups chopped fresh coriander

1 cup chopped fresh mint leaves

8 drops of lemon juice

2 inches ginger

4 teaspoons pani puri masala

4 teaspoons coriander-cumin powder

Salt to taste

4 green chillies, chopped

METHOD

- Combine chopped coriander, mint leaves, lemon juice, ginger, pani puri masala, coriander-cumin powder, salt and green chillies in a blender jar.
- Add four cups of water and blend well.
- Strain and serve chilled.

Recipe courtesy Dr Sarita Davare

Diet Plans: A B C
Portion: 1 glass

Mixed Vegetable Juice

INGREDIENTS

1 inch piece bottle gourd (lauki) or ash gourd (petha), peeled

4 small cucumbers, peeled and roughly chopped

20 fresh spinach leaves

4 medium tomatoes, roughly chopped

8 Indian gooseberries (amla), seeded

8 tablespoons aloe vera juice

1 inch ginger

2 teaspoons lemon juice

A pinch of salt

METHOD

- Blend together the bottle gourd, cucumber, spinach, tomato, gooseberries, aloe vera juice, ginger, lemon juice and salt until smooth.
- Serve chilled.

Recipe courtesy Dr Sarita Davare

Diet Plans: A B C
Portion: 1 glass

Buttermilk Pancakes

INGREDIENTS

1 cup low-fat yogurt buttermilk

1 cup whole-wheat flour (atta)

1 teaspoon baking powder

½ teaspoon soda bicarbonate

A pinch of salt

2 teaspoons oil

1 teaspoon mustard seeds

8-10 curry leaves, chopped

1 inch ginger, chopped

2 green chillies, chopped

METHOD

- Combine the flour, baking powder, soda bicarbonate and salt in a bowl.
- In another bowl, combine the buttermilk and one teaspoon of oil and mix well. Add to the flour mixture and stir quickly to make a smooth batter.
- Heat the remaining oil in a non-stick pan. Add the mustard seeds, curry leaves, ginger and green chilli and sauté until the seeds splutter. Add to the batter and mix well.
- Heat a non-stick tawa. Pour a ladleful of the mixture and spread into a pancake. Cook for two to three minutes on each side.
- Serve hot.

Diet Plans: A B C

Portion: 1½ pancakes

Doodhi Thepla

INGREDIENTS

½ cup grated bottle gourd (doodhi/lauki)

1 cup whole-wheat flour (atta)

½ cup skimmed milk yogurt

Salt to taste

1 teaspoon cumin seeds

½ teaspoon turmeric powder

1 teaspoon red chilli powder

½ tablespoon coriander powder

2 teaspoons oil

METHOD

- Squeeze the grated bottle gourd to remove excess liquid and put into a bowl. Reserve the liquid.
- Add the flour, yogurt, salt, cumin seeds, turmeric powder, chilli powder, coriander powder and two teaspoons oil to the bowl. Add as much of the reserved bottle gourd water as required and knead to make a soft dough.
- Cover the dough with a damp piece of muslin and allow it to rest for ten to fifteen minutes. Divide the dough into eight equal portions and roll out each portion into a thin round (thepla).
- Heat a non-stick tawa and cook the thepla, turning them over and brushing with a little oil, until both sides are evenly golden brown. Serve hot.

Diet Plans: A B

Portion: 2 thepla

Kanchipuram Idli

INGREDIENTS

½ cup rice

¼ cup skinless split black gram (dhuli urad dal)

½ teaspoon fenugreek seeds (methi dana)

½ teaspoon turmeric powder

10 black peppercorns

1 teaspoon split Bengal gram

A pinch of asafoetida (hing)

½ cup low-fat yogurt

1 teaspoon oil

Salt to taste

A few tender banana leaves, cut into squares to line moulds

METHOD

- Soak the rice and split black gram with fenugreek seeds for three to four hours. Drain and grind to a smooth paste with sufficient water to make a thick batter.
- Add the turmeric powder, peppercorns, split Bengal gram, asafoetida, yogurt, oil and salt. Mix well and leave to ferment overnight, or for at least six hours. Whip the batter and adjust the consistency. The batter should be fairly thick.
- Heat sufficient water in a steamer. Line the idli moulds with the banana leaves and pour the batter into them. Place in the steamer and steam for about twenty minutes or until done.
- Carefully remove the idli from the moulds and serve hot.

Diet Plans: A B C
Portion: 2-3 idli

Mooli ka Parantha

INGREDIENTS

1 large white radish (mooli)

1½ cups whole-wheat flour (atta) + for dusting

Salt to taste

2 teaspoons oil

¼ teaspoon red chilli powder

¼ teaspoon carom seeds (ajwain), crushed

1 green chilli, chopped

2 tablespoons fresh coriander, chopped

METHOD

- Separate the leaves from the radish and chop the leaves finely. Grate the radish. Squeeze out the juice from the grated radish. Reserve the radish and the juice separately.
- Mix flour and salt in a bowl. Rub in the oil with your fingertips. Add the reserved radish juice and knead into a soft dough, adding a little water if necessary. Cover with a damp cloth and rest the dough for fifteen minutes.
- Combine grated radish, radish leaves, chilli powder, carom seeds, green chilli and chopped coriander in a bowl. Divide the mixture into six equal portions. Divide the dough into six equal portions. Flatten each portion, making the edges thinner than the centre. Place a portion of the filling in the centre and sprinkle with salt. Gather the edges together and roll into a ball.
- Flatten the ball slightly, and roll out into a parantha on a work surface lightly dusted with flour.
- Heat a non-stick tawa. Place a parantha on the tawa and cook for one minute. Turn over once again and roast until both sides are golden and crisp on the outside. Serve hot.

Diet Plans: A B

Portion: 1½ parantha

Muesli with Fruit

INGREDIENTS

Basic muesli

2 cups porridge oats

¼ cup dried apricots, chopped

8 almonds, sliced

2 tablespoons black currants

1 cup cornflakes

To serve

¼ cup dried figs, chopped

Fresh fruit (such as strawberries, bananas, apples, grapes), chopped

Cold skimmed milk or low-fat yogurt

METHOD

- For the basic muesli, dry-roast the porridge oats.
- Combine the roasted oats, apricots, almonds, black currants and cornflakes, in a bowl. Store in an airtight container.
- To serve, place a few tablespoons of muesli in a bowl. Add the chopped figs and chopped fresh fruit.
- Pour the milk over the muesli and serve. You may heat the milk if desired.
- If serving the muesli with yogurt, add the figs, fresh fruit and yogurt to the muesli. Mix and let stand for about five to ten minutes before serving.

Diet Plans: A B

Portion: 1 bowl/1½ katori

Set Dosa

INGREDIENTS

1 cup rice

½ cup beaten rice (poha)

¼ teaspoon fenugreek seeds (methi dana)

Salt to taste

1 cup low-fat yogurt

2 teaspoons oil

METHOD

- Wash and soak the rice and fenugreek seeds in two cups of warm water for about two hours.
- Soak the beaten rice in a little water for about five minutes. Grind the rice and fenugreek seeds along with the beaten rice and salt to make a smooth, thick batter.
- Transfer to a bowl, add the yogurt and mix well and leave the batter in a warm place to ferment overnight. Heat a non-stick tawa and grease it lightly.
- For each dosa, pour a ladleful of batter onto the tawa, but do not spread it. The batter will set in a thick round. Drizzle a little oil all around the dosa and cover it with a lid. Cook until the underside is done and very light brown. Serve hot.

Chef's Tip

For added flavour, add green chillies and ginger while grinding the rice.

Diet Plan: A
Portion: 2 dosai

Sooji Pancakes

INGREDIENTS

½ cup coarse semolina (sooji)

2 tablespoons gram flour (besan)

Salt to taste

½ teaspoon cumin seeds

A pinch of asafoetida (hing)

1 green chilli, chopped

3 tablespoons skimmed milk yogurt

¼ teaspoon fruit salt

2 teaspoons oil

1 medium tomato, finely chopped

2 tablespoons chopped fresh coriander

METHOD

- Combine the semolina, gram flour, salt, cumin seeds, asafoetida, green chilli, yogurt and sufficient water to make a smooth batter. Leave the batter to rest for fifteen to twenty minutes.
- Add the fruit salt to the batter and mix.
- Heat a non-stick pan. Drizzle a little oil on the pan; spread a ladleful of batter to make a slightly thick four-inch round pancake. Cook on medium heat. Sprinkle a little tomato, and chopped coriander over it. Cover and cook for three to four minutes.
- Uncover the pan, drizzle a little oil all around and cook until the underside is crisp. Serve hot.

Diet Plans: A B

Portion: 2 pancakes

Vegetable and Oatmeal Upma

INGREDIENTS

1 carrot, chopped

3-4 French beans, chopped

½ cup green peas

1 cup oatmeal

2 teaspoons oil

½ teaspoon mustard seeds

1 teaspoon split Bengal gram

½ teaspoon cumin seeds

A pinch of asafoetida (hing)

1 inch ginger, finely chopped

2 green chillies, slit

1 onion, finely chopped

4-6 curry leaves

Salt to taste

METHOD

- Dry-roast oats in a non-stick pan for two minutes and set aside.
- Heat oil in another non-stick pan and add mustard seeds. When they begin to splutter, add split Bengal gram, cumin seeds and sauté until they change colour.
- Add asafoetida, chopped ginger and green chillies, and sauté for a few seconds. Add onion, carrot, French beans, green peas, curry leaves and salt to taste, and sauté for half a minute.
- Add one and a half cups of water and cook until the vegetables are tender. Add oatmeal and mix well. Reduce heat and cook until the oatmeal is done. Serve hot.

Diet Plans: A B

Portion: 1 bowl/1½ katori

Poached Eggs on Vegetables

INGREDIENTS

8 egg whites

20 spinach leaves, chopped

16-20 mushrooms, chopped

2 medium onions, chopped

Salt to taste

2 tablespoons white vinegar

4 whole-wheat bread slices

2 slices chicken salami, chopped (optional)

METHOD

- Heat three-fourth cup of water in a non-stick pan.
- Add spinach, mushrooms, onion and salt and cook for three to four minutes, or until most of the moisture has been absorbed. Divide into four equal portions.
- Heat three cups of water in another non-stick pan. Place a metal egg ring in the centre. Add half a tablespoon of vinegar. Slide 2 egg whites into the ring and cook on low heat. Cut bread into thick slices. Place a slice on the serving plate. Place one portion of vegetables on it.
- Gently separate the eggs from the ring with a knife and remove the ring carefully. Carefully lift the eggs with a slotted spoon and place over the vegetables on the bread slice. Place the chicken salami over the eggs and serve immediately.

Diet Plans: A C

Portion: 1 slice bread with 2 egg whites and vegetables

Scrambled Eggs with Mushrooms and Peas

INGREDIENTS

8 egg whites, beaten well

10-12 fresh button mushrooms, sliced

½ cup green peas, boiled

2 teaspoons butter

2 large onions, finely chopped

Salt to taste

2 large tomatoes, finely chopped

2 tablespoons chopped fresh coriander

½ teaspoon white pepper powder

METHOD

- Heat the butter in a non-stick pan. Add the onions and sauté until the onions turn soft.
- Add the mushrooms and sprinkle some salt. Cook on high heat until the moisture dries up.
- Add the peas and tomatoes and sauté for a few seconds.
- Add the beaten egg whites and stir continuously on medium heat until the eggs scramble. Add the chopped coriander, salt and white pepper powder.
- Mix well and serve immediately.

Diet Plans: A B
Portion: 2 egg whites

Oriental Mixed Vegetable Soup

INGREDIENTS

½ cup sweet corn kernels (makai ke dane)

150 grams cream-style sweet corn

¼ small cabbage, chopped

¼ medium carrot, chopped

100 grams bean curd (tofu), cut into ½-inch pieces

2 teaspoons oil

4-5 cups Vegetable Stock (page 307)

Salt to taste

¼ teaspoon white-pepper powder

½ teaspoon sugar

1 tablespoon cornflour, mixed in ½ cup water

1 spring onion, green part only, chopped

METHOD

- Heat oil in a non-stick wok; add the corn kernels, cabbage and carrot and stir-fry for two minutes. Stir in vegetable stock and bring to a boil.
- Mix in the cream-style corn and continue to cook for two to three minutes.
- Add salt, white pepper powder and sugar, and stir to mix.
- Add bean curd and stir in the cornflour mixture. Cook, stirring continuously, for one minute or until the soup thickens.
- Serve piping hot, garnished with spring onion greens.

Diet Plans: A B

Portion: 1 bowl (1½ katori)

Jau aur Subziyon ka Shorba

INGREDIENTS

¼ cup pearl barley (jau)

3-4 French beans, finely chopped

½ medium carrot, finely chopped

3 small broccoli florets, finely chopped

2 small cauliflower florets, finely chopped

3 teaspoons oil

8-10 garlic cloves, chopped

½ inch ginger, grated

1 small onion, chopped

¼ tablespoon black peppercorns

2 bay leaves

Salt to taste

4-5 fresh coriander sprigs

METHOD

- Wash the barley well and drain thoroughly.
- Heat one teaspoon oil in a non-stick pan; add the barley and sauté until lightly browned and dry. Transfer to a bowl, add one cup of water and leave to soak overnight or for atleast six hours.
- When ready to cook, heat two teaspoons oil in a deep non-stick pan. Add the garlic and ginger and sauté for a minute.

- Add the onion and sauté on medium heat until the onion turns translucent.
- Drain the barley and add it to the pan; sauté for two to three minutes. Add the peppercorns and bay leaves and sauté for a minute longer.
- Reserve a small quantity of the French beans, carrot and broccoli and add the rest to the pan along with the cauliflower and salt, and sauté for two minutes.
- Add the coriander sprigs and six cups of water and bring to a boil on high heat.
- Lower the heat and simmer for at least twenty to twenty-five minutes, or until the broth is reduced to half its original quantity.
- Strain the soup into another deep non-stick pan. Add the reserved French beans, carrot and broccoli and cook for five to seven minutes.
- Serve piping hot.

Diet Plans: A B

Portion: 1 bowl (1½ katori)

Pepper Rasam

INGREDIENTS

10-12 black peppercorns, coarsely powdered

3 tablespoons split pigeon peas (arhar dal/ toovar dal), soaked

1 teaspoon split Bengal gram

1 teaspoon skinless split black gram (dhuli urad dal)

6-7 dried red chillies

¼ teaspoon fenugreek seeds

½ teaspoon cumin seeds

¾ teaspoon mustard seeds

1 teaspoon coriander seeds

1 teaspoon oil

3 garlic cloves, crushed

10 curry leaves

Salt to taste

¼ teaspoon turmeric powder

2 tablespoons tamarind pulp

1½ teaspoons grated jaggery

Seasoning

1 teaspoon oil

½ teaspoon mustard seeds

2 dried red chillies

¼ teaspoon asafoetida (hing)

10 curry leaves

METHOD

- Pressure-cook the pigeon peas in one cup of water until the pressure is released three times (three whistles).
- Remove the lid when the pressure reduces completely and mash the dal. Set aside.
- Dry-roast the Bengal gram and black gram, red chillies, fenugreek seeds, cumin seeds, half a teaspoon of mustard seeds and coriander seeds. Grind together to a powder.

- Heat the oil in a deep non-stick pan and add garlic, remaining mustard seeds, peppercorns and curry leaves.
- When the mustard starts to splutter, add the mashed dal, the roasted spice powder mixed with a little water, salt, turmeric powder, tamarind pulp and jaggery. Blend well and add five cups of water. Bring to a boil.
- Simmer on low heat for ten to fifteen minutes. Strain the mixture through a piece of muslin.
- For the seasoning, heat oil in a non-stick pan. Add mustard seeds; and when they splutter add red chillies, asafoetida and curry leaves.
- Pour over the rasam and serve hot.

Diet Plans: A B C

Portion: 1 bowl (1½ katori)

Roasted Red Pepper Soup

INGREDIENTS

8 medium red capsicums

2 medium onions, chopped

12 garlic cloves, chopped

1 tablespoon whole-wheat flour (atta)

8 cups Vegetable Stock (page 307)

4-5 fresh basil leaves (tulsi)

Salt to taste

1 teaspoon sugar or equivalent sugar substitute

5-6 black peppercorns, crushed

4 tablespoons lemon juice

METHOD

- Prick capsicums using a fork and roast them directly over an open flame on low heat until lightly charred. Plunge them into cold water, remove skin and chop them roughly.
- Place onions and garlic in a non-stick pan and roast on medium heat for a minute. Add flour and continue to roast for another minute until light brown and fragrant.
- Add one cup of vegetable stock, the capsicums and two to three fresh basil leaves. Stir and bring to a boil. Cover and simmer for three to four minutes. Cool and blend to a smooth purée.
- Transfer to a thick-bottomed non-stick pan, add the remaining stock and bring to a boil. Reduce heat, add salt, sugar and crushed black peppercorns. Simmer for two to three minutes. Stir in the lemon juice and pour into soup bowls. Serve hot, garnished with remaining basil.

Diet Plans: A B C

Portion: 1 bowl (1½ katori)

Tofu, Moong Dal and Spinach Soup

INGREDIENTS

8 teaspoons grated bean curd (tofu)

4 tablespoons skinless split green gram (dhuli moong dal), soaked for 5-10 minutes

2 cups finely chopped spinach

4 cups Vegetable Stock (page 307)

4 small onions, chopped

A pinch of black pepper powder

½ teaspoon salt

METHOD

- Heat a pressure cooker and add the green gram, spinach, one and a half cups of vegetable stock or water and onion. Pressure-cook on medium heat until the pressure is released four times (four whistles), or until the ingredients turn mushy.
- When the pressure reduces completely, remove the lid and transfer the contents to a blender jar. Blend the mixture into a smooth purée. Transfer the purée into a deep non-stick pan.
- Add the remaining stock, pepper powder, salt and tofu, stir to mix and bring to a boil.
- Serve piping hot.

Recipe courtesy Dr Sarita Davare

Diet Plans: A B C

Portion: 1 bowl (1½ katori)

Tomato Basil Shorba

INGREDIENTS

6 medium tomatoes, roughly chopped

3-4 basil leaves (tulsi)

7 garlic cloves

1 inch cinnamon

1 black cardamom

½ tablespoon black peppercorns

1 tablespoon cumin seeds

2 dried red chillies

½ cup chopped fresh coriander stems

1 teaspoon oil

½ teaspoon red chilli powder (deghi mirch)

2 tablespoons gram flour

½ tablespoon lemon juice

Basil pesto

6-8 fresh basil leaves (tulsi)

3 garlic cloves

2 cashew nuts

2 teaspoons olive oil

METHOD

- Combine the tomatoes, basil, garlic, cinnamon, cardamom, peppercorns, cumin seeds, red chillies, coriander stems, five cups of water and oil in a deep non-stick pan and boil for ten to twelve minutes.
- Add chilli powder and mix. Take the pan off the heat and strain the mixture into another deep non-stick pan.
- Add one cup of water and boil for five minutes.

- Roast gram flour in another small non-stick pan until fragrant.
- Add half a cup of water and mix well. Add this to the shorba and cook for five minutes.
- To make the pesto, grind together basil leaves, garlic and cashew nuts with oil to a smooth paste.
- Stir the lemon juice into the shorba. Serve hot, topped with a dollop of pesto.

Diet Plans: A B

Portion: 1 bowl (1½ katori)

Spinach and Baby Corn Soup

INGREDIENTS

40 fresh spinach leaves, chopped

8 pieces baby corn, finely chopped

4 medium onions, chopped

4 cups Vegetable Stock (page 307)

1 teaspoon salt

A large pinch of black pepper powder

METHOD

- Heat a deep non-stick pan. Add the onions, baby corn and spinach and sauté until the leaves wilt.
- Stir in the vegetable stock and bring to a boil.
- Remove the mixture from heat and cool to room temperature. Blend to a smooth purée and transfer back into the pan.
- Add the salt and pepper powder, mix well and bring to a boil.
- Serve piping hot.

Recipe courtesy Dr Sarita Davare

Diet Plans: A B C

Portion: 1 bowl (1½ katori)

Minestrone Soup with Chicken

INGREDIENTS

12-15 small ripe red tomatoes

½ cup minced chicken

1 teaspoon olive oil

1¼ tablespoons chopped garlic

1 medium carrot, cut into small pieces

2 tablespoons whole-wheat macaroni

3 cups Chicken Stock (page 307)

Salt to taste

1 teaspoon crushed peppercorns

A few fresh basil leaves (tulsi)

1 teaspoon grated Parmesan cheese, to serve (optional)

METHOD

- Score the base of the tomatoes and blanch them in plenty of hot water for two to three minutes and transfer them immediately to a bowl of cold water.
- Peel, halve and remove seeds. Purée the tomatoes in a blender. Divide chicken mince into small equal portions and shape into balls.
- Heat olive oil in a non-stick pan. Add garlic, carrot, macaroni and three-fourth cup of water. Stir in the tomato purée along with chicken stock. Add salt and crushed peppercorns, stir again, cover and cook until it comes to a boil.
- Add chicken mince balls and cook, removing the scum that rises to the surface. Cook until macaroni is just cooked. Tear basil leaves and add to the soup. Ladle the soup into serving bowls, sprinkle Parmesan cheese on top and serve hot.

Diet Plan: A

Portion: 1 bowl (1½ katori)

Mexican Chicken Hot Pot

INGREDIENTS

200 grams boneless chicken, cut into 1-inch cubes

3 tablespoons whole-wheat flour

¼ cup red kidney beans (rajma), soaked overnight

Salt to taste

2 medium onions

3 teaspoons oil

4-5 garlic cloves, finely chopped

6 cups Chicken Stock (page 307)

1 small potato, cut into ½-inch cubes

1 teaspoon Tabasco sauce

1 teaspoon paprika powder

¼ teaspoon dried thyme

2 medium tomatoes, seeded and cut into ½-inch cubes

1 medium green capsicum, cut into ½-inch cubes

¼ teaspoon black pepper powder

METHOD

- Dust the chicken cubes with flour and keep aside.
- Drain the kidney beans, add three-fourth cup of water and salt and pressure cook until pressure is released five to six times (five to six whistles).

- Finely chop one onion and cut the other into half-inch cubes. Heat two teaspoons oil in a deep non-stick pan. Add garlic and chopped onion and sauté until light brown.
- Add chicken and sauté until nicely browned.
- Add chicken stock and bring to a boil. Add the kidney beans and simmer until the mutton is three-fourth cooked.
- Add the potato and simmer for ten minutes. Add the Tabasco sauce, paprika and thyme and simmer for a minute. Add the tomatoes and simmer for five more minutes. Remove from the heat.
- In a separate non-stick frying pan, sauté the capsicum and onion cubes in the remaining oil and add to the soup.
- Season with salt and pepper powder and serve hot.

Diet Plan: A

Portion: 1 bowl (1½ katori)

Murgh Yakhni

INGREDIENTS

100 grams boneless chicken breast (fat removed), boiled and cut into ½-inch cubes

1 teaspoon oil

2 medium onions, chopped

2 tablespoons low-fat yogurt, whisked

1 tablespoon whole-wheat flour

2 garlic cloves, chopped

1 teaspoon fennel seeds (saunf)

8 black peppercorns

2 black cardamoms

4 green cardamoms

2 bay leaves

3 cups Chicken Stock (page 307)

Salt to taste

2 inches ginger, chopped

METHOD

- Heat oil in a deep non-stick pan; add onions and sauté until golden.
- Stir in the yogurt and cook until the moisture evaporates. Add flour, and sauté for a couple of minutes.
- Add garlic, fennel seeds, peppercorns, black cardamoms, green cardamoms and bay leaves, and mix well. Add chicken stock and stir, ensuring there are no lumps. Simmer on low heat for fifteen minutes. Add salt and ginger and mix. Cook for five minutes until the mixture reduces slightly.
- Strain into soup bowls, add the chicken and serve hot.

Diet Plans: A C

Portion: 1 bowl (1½ katori)

Murgh Pudina Shorba

INGREDIENTS

350 grams boneless chicken (fat removed), cut into ½-inch cubes

25-30 fresh mint leaves, roughly chopped

2 teaspoons oil

1 teaspoon cumin seeds

1 medium onion, chopped

1 garlic clove, chopped

¼ teaspoon red chilli flakes

½ teaspoon cinnamon powder

1 green cardamom

2 medium tomatoes, peeled, seeded and roughly chopped

½ cup chickpeas (Kabuli chana), boiled

A few saffron threads

Salt to taste

½ cup skimmed milk yogurt, whisked

METHOD

- Heat the oil in a pressure cooker; add the cumin seeds and sauté until they begin to change colour. Add the onion and sauté until translucent. Add the garlic, chilli flakes, mint leaves and chicken. Continue to sauté for a few seconds.
- Add the cinnamon powder and cardamom and sauté for two more minutes. Add the tomatoes, chickpeas, saffron, salt and six cups of water and bring to a boil. Pressure-cook for around eight to ten minutes until pressure is released 3 times (3 whistles).
- Remove the lid when the pressure has reduced completely; stir in the yogurt and cook over low heat for two to three minutes. Serve hot.

Diet Plan: A

Portion: 1 bowl (1½ katori)

Hot and Sour Shredded Chicken Soup

INGREDIENTS

4 fresh red chillies, seeded and sliced diagonally

2 lemongrass roots, sliced

2-3 lime leaves

2 lemons

200 grams boneless, skinless chicken breasts, finely chopped

4 cups Chicken Stock (page 307)

8-10 fresh spinach leaves, finely chopped

2 inches galangal, sliced

Salt to taste

A pinch of sugar

1 teaspoon fish sauce

METHOD

- Heat chicken stock in a deep non-stick pan. Add lemongrass roots and galangal. Bruise lime leaves and add to the pan.
- Add two red chillies to the pan along with salt and sugar.
- Slice one lemon into thin slices. Reserve a few slices to garnish, and add the rest to the pan.
- Boil the stock for five to ten minutes. Strain into a bowl and pour the strained stock back into the pan and place on heat. Add chicken along with fish sauce, spinach and red chillies and cook until the chicken is tender.
- Stir in the juice of the remaining lemon. Take the pan off the heat and pour the soup into a serving bowl.
- Garnish with reserved lemon slices and serve hot.

Diet Plans: A C

Portion: 1 bowl (1½ katori)

Chickpea and Red Capsicum Salad

INGREDIENTS

2 cups boiled chickpeas, drained

2 small red capsicums, roasted

12 black olives, stoned

1 tablespoon chopped fresh parsley

Dressing

1 teaspoon oil

1 teaspoon grated orange rind

2 tablespoons fresh orange juice

2-3 garlic cloves, crushed

Salt to taste

4-6 black peppercorns, crushed

METHOD

- Keep the boiled chickpeas warm. Mix together all the ingredients for the dressing.
- Toss the chickpeas while they are still warm into the dressing. Set aside to cool.
- Peel the roasted capsicums. Cut in half, remove the core and seeds and slice thinly. Add the capsicums, olives and half the parsley to the chickpeas.
- Transfer the salad to a serving bowl or platter, and garnish with the remaining parsley.

Chef's Tip

To remove the skins of the capsicums easily, place the hot roasted capsicums in a plastic bag for a few minutes, or in a bowl covered tightly with cling film–the steam will loosen the skins.

Diet Plans: A B C

Portion: 1 bowl (1½ katori)

Crunchy Celery, Cucumber and Pomegranate Medley

INGREDIENTS

3 celery stalks, trimmed and chopped

2 small cucumbers, chopped

¾ cup fresh pomegranate seeds

¾ cup halved seedless grapes

A few lettuce leaves

Dressing

½ cup low-fat yogurt, whisked

¾ teaspoon honey

¾ teaspoon mustard paste

Salt to taste

Black pepper powder to taste

METHOD

- Place the celery, cucumber, pomegranate and grapes in a large salad bowl.
- Place in a refrigerator to chill thoroughly for at least half an hour.
- Mix together all the ingredients for the dressing.
- Just before serving, pour the dressing over the salad and toss well to mix.
- Serve on a bed of lettuce.

Diet Plans: A B C
Portion: 1 bowl (1½ katori)

Fruit and Capsicum Kachumber

INGREDIENTS

2 medium apples, cored and sliced thinly

2 medium oranges

12-15 seedless green grapes, halved

12-15 seedless black grapes, halved

1 medium green capsicum, cut into thin strips

1 tablespoons lemon juice

1 medium cucumber, sliced thinly

2 medium tomatoes, seeded and cut into thin strips

2 spring onions, sliced thinly

Dressing

1 tablespoon chopped fresh coriander

8-10 fresh mint leaves, roughly torn

2 green chillies, chopped

1½ teaspoons chaat masala

1 tablespoon lemon juice

Salt to taste

METHOD

- Sprinkle one tablespoon of lemon juice over the apple slices to prevent oxidation.
- Peel the oranges and separate the segments. Remove the seeds and white membrane from each segment, and cut each one in half.
- For the dressing, mix together the chopped coriander, mint leaves, green chillies, chaat masala, lemon juice and salt.
- Toss the fruit and vegetables in the dressing and serve chilled.

Diet Plans: A B C

Portion: 1 bowl (1½ katori)

Moong aur Moth ka Anokha Salad

INGREDIENTS

½ cup sprouted whole green gram (moong)

½ cup sprouted brown gram (moth/matki)

½ level teaspoon salt

1 green chilli, finely chopped

1 medium onion, cut into ½-inch cubes, layers separated

1 medium green capsicum, cut into ½-inch cubes

1 medium cucumber, cut into ½-inch cubes

2 medium tomatoes, cut into ½-inch pieces

¼ medium apple, thinly sliced

5-6 freshly crushed black peppercorns

1 tablespoon lemon juice

METHOD

- Place the green gram and brown gram sprouts in two separate bowls.
- Add salt and half a cup of water to each bowl and cook the sprouts in the microwave for two minutes on HIGH. Drain and transfer both into a deep bowl.
- Add the chilli, onion, capsicum, cucumber, tomatoes and apple, and toss to mix.
- Add the crushed peppercorns and lemon juice and mix well. Chill and serve.

Diet Plans: A B C

Portion: 1 bowl (1½ katori)

Mosambi Salad

INGREDIENTS

2 medium sweet limes (mosambi)

2 medium cucumbers, peeled and chopped

2 medium tomatoes, seeded and chopped

2 small onions, chopped

1 teaspoon chaat masala

½ teaspoon salt

4 teaspoons yogurt

METHOD

- Peel the sweet limes and separate the segments. Remove the seeds and white membrane from each segment, and cut each one in half.
- Combine the sweet lime, cucumber, tomato and onion in a bowl.
- Add the chaat masala, salt and yogurt and toss to mix.
- Serve chilled.

Recipe courtesy Dr Sarita Davare

Diet Plans: A B C

Portion: 1 bowl (1½ katori)

Pomegranate, Cucumber and Tomato Salad

INGREDIENTS

½ cup fresh pomegranate seeds

2 medium cucumbers, peeled and diced

2 medium tomatoes, seeded and diced

½ teaspoon chaat masala

A pinch of salt

4 teaspoons yogurt

METHOD

- Combine the pomegranate, cucumber and tomato in a bowl.
- Add the chaat masala, salt and yogurt and toss to mix.
- Serve chilled.

Recipe courtesy Dr Sarita Davare

Diet Plans: A B C

Portion: 1 bowl (1½ katori)

Rajma Salad

INGREDIENTS

1 cup boiled kidney beans (rajma)

1 medium tomato, seeded and chopped

2 spring onions with greens, chopped

1 tablespoon lemon juice

½ teaspoon salt

A pinch of black pepper powder

METHOD

- Combine the kidney beans, tomato and spring onion in a bowl.
- Add the lemon juice, salt and pepper powder and toss to mix.
- Serve chilled.

Recipe courtesy Dr Sarita Davare

Diet Plans: A B C

Portion: 1 cup (1 katori)

Sprouted Fenugreek Salad

INGREDIENTS

½ cup fresh fenugreek seeds (methi dana)

¾ cup chopped fresh coriander

1 medium tomato, seeded and chopped fine

½ tablespoon lemon juice

A pinch of salt

METHOD

- Soak the fenugreek seeds in half a cup of water for eight hours.
- Drain, transfer to a piece of muslin, gather the corners of the muslin and seal with a knot. Set aside for twenty-four hours, or until the seeds sprout.
- Place the sprouted fenugreek seeds in a bowl. Add the chopped coriander, tomato, lemon juice and salt, and mix well.
- Serve chilled.

Recipe courtesy Dr Sarita Davare

Diet Plans: A B C

Portion: 1 cup (1 katori)

Apple, Barley and Pumpkin Seed Salad

INGREDIENTS

1 medium red apple

¼ cup fresh apple juice

½ cup pearl barley

2 teaspoons pumpkin seeds

1 tablespoon lemon juice

Salt to taste

2 teaspoons extra-virgin olive oil

10-15 fresh mint leaves

2-3 fresh parsley sprigs

4-5 fresh coriander sprigs

¼ teaspoon black pepper powder

Few iceberg lettuce leaves

Few lollo rosso lettuce leaves

1 teaspoon honey

METHOD

- Slice the apples thickly, core and cut into large pieces and put them into a bowl. Stir in half a tablespoon lemon juice to prevent oxidation.
- Toast the barley in a non-stick pan for two minutes. Add one and a half cups of water and cook barley until soft. Drain and add to the bowl.
- Heat another non-stick pan and lightly toast the pumpkin seeds. Leave to cool. Add salt, apple juice, olive oil and remaining lemon juice to the barley and apples, and mix.
- Roughly chop fresh mint, parsley and coriander. Add the chopped herbs to the bowl and season with the pepper powder. Roughly tear the lettuce leaves, and add to the bowl. Add the honey and pumpkin seeds and toss well to mix.
- Transfer into a serving bowl and serve immediately.

Diet Plans: A B

Portion: 1 bowl (1½ katori)

Quinoa, Pomegranate and Spinach Salad

INGREDIENTS

¼ cup cooked quinoa

¼ cup fresh pomegranate seeds

2 cups baby spinach

1 small cucumber, peeled and diced

½ medium apple, chopped

1 small onion, chopped

Dressing

3 teaspoons extra-virgin olive oil

1 teaspoon apple cider vinegar

Salt to taste

¼ teaspoon black pepper powder

¼ teaspoon Italian seasoning

METHOD

- In a bowl, combine the quinoa, pomegranate, baby spinach, cucumber, apple and onion and toss to mix.
- To make the dressing, in a small bowl, combine the olive oil, vinegar, salt, pepper powder and Italian seasoning and stir to mix.
- Pour the dressing over the salad and serve.

Note: *Quinoa is pronounced 'keen-wah'.*

Diet Plans: A B

Portion: 1 bowl (1½ katori)

Kale and Mint Tabouleh

INGREDIENTS

1 cup roughly chopped kale

¼ cup chopped fresh mint leaves

¼ cup broken wheat, washed and soaked

Salt to taste

1 medium tomato, finely chopped

1 medium onion, finely chopped

3 tablespoons chopped fresh coriander

Juice of 1 lemon

METHOD

- Heat sufficient water in a deep non-stick pan; add the salt and broken wheat, mix and cook until tender. Drain, transfer into a bowl and set aside to cool.
- When completely cooled, add the chopped kale, mint, tomato, onion, chopped coriander and lemon juice; toss to mix.
- Serve immediately.

Diet Plans: A B

Portion: 1 bowl (1½ katori)

Warm Quinoa Salad with Grilled Tofu

INGREDIENTS

½ cup quinoa

100 grams bean curd (tofu), cut into ½-inch thick slices

2 teaspoons olive oil

1½ cups Vegetable Stock (page 307)

Salt to taste

Crushed black peppercorns to taste

½ medium green capsicum, cut into ½-inch pieces

½ medium onion, cut into ½-inch pieces

4 pickled jalapeño slices roughly chopped

4-5 fresh curly parsley sprigs, roughly chopped

Juice of ½ lemon

METHOD

- Heat one teaspoon olive oil in a deep non-stick pan; add the quinoa and sauté until golden.
- Add the vegetable stock, salt and crushed peppercorns, and mix well. Cover and cook until the quinoa is tender.
- Heat half a teaspoon olive oil in a non-stick grill pan; add the onion, capsicum, salt and crushed peppercorns and sauté until soft. Transfer into a large bowl.
- Place the grill pan back on heat; add the remaining olive oil.

- Place the tofu on the hot grill pan; sprinkle salt and pepper and grill, turning over, until grill marks appear on both sides.
- Add the quinoa, pickled jalapeños, parsley and lemon juice to the onion and capsicum, and toss to mix.
- Transfer the salad to a serving plate, top with grilled tofu slices and serve immediately.

Diet Plans: A B

Portion: 1 bowl (1½ katori)

Salade Niçoise

INGREDIENTS

1 head of iceberg lettuce

2 medium potatoes

15 French beans

4 medium tomatoes, quartered

4 hard-boiled eggs, whites only, quartered

1 teaspoon vinegar

1 teaspoon olive oil

A pinch of salt

¼ teaspoon crushed black peppercorns

1 teaspoon chopped fresh mixed herbs

10 black olives, stoned

METHOD

- Tear the lettuce into bite-size pieces and soak in chilled water.
- Boil, peel and dice the potatoes. Blanch the French beans and cut into two-inch pieces.
- Place the potatoes, French beans, tomatoes and egg whites in a large bowl. Toss once to mix.
- Mix vinegar, olive oil, salt, crushed peppercorns and mixed herbs in a bowl.
- Pour the dressing over, and using two forks, carefully toss the vegetables until they are thoroughly coated.
- Drain the lettuce leaves and arrange on a large, shallow serving platter.
- Spoon the salad onto the lettuce leaves and garnish with black olives. Serve immediately.

Diet Plans: A B

Portion: 1 bowl (1½ katori)

Spicy Mexican Chicken and Corn Salad with Beans

INGREDIENTS

2 cooked chicken sausages, cut into ½-inch pieces

½ cup sweet corn kernels (makai ke daane), boiled

½ cup boiled red kidney beans (rajma), drained

1 small onion, cut into ½-inch pieces

1 small green capsicum, cut into ½-inch pieces

5-6 tortilla chips, crushed

Dressing

1 tablespoons chilli sauce

½ tablespoon tomato ketchup

½ tablespoon lemon juice

1 fresh red chilli, cut into thin slivers

A pinch of salt

METHOD

- Place the chicken sausages, corn, kidney beans, onion and capsicum in a large bowl. Toss lightly to mix.
- For the dressing, mix together the chilli sauce, tomato ketchup, lemon juice, red chilli and salt in a small bowl.
- Just before serving, spoon the dressing over the salad and toss well to mix.
- Serve sprinkled with crushed tortilla chips.

***Note:** For a vegetarian version of this salad, replace chicken sausage with a hundred grams of tofu.*

Diet Plan: A

Portion: 1 bowl (1½ katori) with ½ sliced sausage

Grilled Chicken and Mushroom Salad

INGREDIENTS

2 (150 grams each) boneless, skinless chicken breasts

6 large fresh button mushrooms, sliced thickly

Salt to taste

½ teaspoon black pepper powder

½ teaspoon mustard paste

½ teaspoon garlic paste

2 teaspoons oil

1 medium yellow capsicum

1 medium red capsicum

6 black olives, stoned and sliced

½ head of iceberg lettuce, roughly torn

Dressing

1 teaspoon olive oil

1½ tablespoons lemon juice

7-8 black peppercorns, crushed

1 teaspoon powdered sugar, or equivalent sugar substitute

Salt to taste

METHOD

- Marinate the chicken breasts in a mixture of salt, pepper powder, mustard paste and garlic paste for twenty minutes.
- Mix together all the ingredients for the dressing in a bowl.

- Grill the chicken breasts in a non-stick grill pan for five to six minutes on each side. Cool and slice. Brush the mushrooms with oil and grill for two minutes. Cut into quarters.
- Brush the yellow and red capsicums with oil and grill for ten minutes, turning them over once or twice to cook evenly. Cut in half, remove the seeds and slice lengthways.
- Place the chicken, mushrooms, capsicums, olives and lettuce in a large bowl.
- Pour the dressing over the salad and toss well to mix. Serve immediately.

Diet Plans: A C

Portion: 1 bowl (1½ katori) with 6 slices chicken

Grilled Chicken and Fruit Salad

INGREDIENTS

200 grams skinless, boneless chicken breast

75 grams seedless green grapes, peeled and halved

1 pear (naspati), peeled, cored and sliced

Salt to taste

2 teaspoons lemon juice

25 grams walnut (akhrot) halves

4 iceberg lettuce leaves, shredded

2 celery stalks, chopped

1 red capsicum, seeded and sliced

Dressing

4 tablespoons low-fat yogurt

2 tablespoons grated cucumber

1 teaspoon grated onion

½ teaspoon chopped fresh thyme, or ¼ teaspoon dried thyme

Salt to taste

Black pepper powder to taste

METHOD

- Marinate the chicken breast with salt and lemon juice for about half an hour. Grill in a non-stick grill pan until both sides are evenly cooked and golden. Set aside to cool. Cut into strips.
- In a large bowl, combine the chicken strips with the grapes, pear, walnuts, lettuce, celery and capsicum.
- In a separate bowl, combine the yogurt, cucumber, onion, thyme, salt and pepper powder.
- Just before serving, spoon the dressing over the salad ingredients and toss well to mix.

Diet Plans: A C

Portion: 1 bowl (1½ katori) with 6 slices chicken

Corn and Sprouted Bean Burritos

INGREDIENTS

¼ cup cooked or tinned corn kernels

½ cup sprouted whole green gram (ankurit moong), blanched

4 home-made whole-wheat flour (atta) tortillas

2 tablespoons grated mozzarella cheese

Salt to taste

5-6 black peppercorns, crushed

½ tablespoon lemon juice

1 small tomato, chopped

½ cup shredded lettuce

1 spring onion, chopped

1 green chilli, chopped

2 tablespoons ready-made spicy salsa

METHOD

- Preheat the oven to 200°C/400°F/Gas Mark 6.
- Mix together cheese, salt, crushed peppercorns, lemon juice and sprouted gram in a bowl.
- In another bowl, mix together tomato, lettuce and spring onion. Add corn kernels and green chilli and mix. Place the tortillas on a plate. Arrange cheese and gram mixture, and corn and tomato mixture in layers on the tortillas. Top with salsa and fold each tortilla over.
- Arrange in a baking dish and bake in the preheated oven for twenty minutes. Serve hot.

Diet Plans: A B

Portion: 1 burrito

Kachche Kele ki Pav Bhaji

INGREDIENTS

1 unripe banana, boiled, peeled and mashed

4 whole-wheat pavs

½ medium green capsicum, finely chopped

3 tablespoons chopped fresh coriander + for garnishing

2 medium tomatoes, finely chopped

¼ cup green peas

Salt to taste

2 teaspoons oil

1¼ teaspoons cumin seeds

¼ teaspoon turmeric powder

1 teaspoon red chilli powder

2 teaspoons garam masala powder

2 teaspoons pav bhaji masala

1 teaspoon butter

METHOD

- Heat oil in a non-stick pan; add cumin seeds and sauté until brown.
- Add capsicum and sauté for a minute. Add salt, mix well and add mashed banana. Mix well and sauté for a minute.
- Add three tablespoons chopped coriander and mix well.

- Add turmeric powder, chilli powder, garam masala powder and pav bhaji masala. Mix well and cook for two minutes.
- Add tomato, green peas and two tablespoons water.
- Mix well, adjust salt and cook for three to four minutes, mashing the vegetables as they cook. Remove from heat and transfer to a serving bowl.
- Slit pavs horizontally without cutting through. Roast them on a non-stick tawa with butter until crisp.
- Garnish bhaji with chopped coriander and serve hot with pavs.

Diet Plan: A
B if pav is made from jowar ka atta
C if the pav is omitted

Portion: 1 pav and 1 cup (1 katori) bhaji

Spicy Corn on the Cob

INGREDIENTS

2 pieces American corn on the cob, halved

Salt to taste

1½ teaspoons red chilli powder

4 teaspoons lemon juice

2 teaspoons oil

METHOD

- Mix together salt, chilli powder and lemon juice in a bowl.
- Add oil and mix well. Rub the mixture over the corn and leave for a few minutes.
- Heat a non-stick grill pan on high heat.
- Place the marinated corn on the grill pan and grill, turning the corn, until it is done on all sides.
- Remove from heat and serve immediately.

Diet Plans: A B

Portion: ½ corn on the cob

Kale Chips

INGREDIENTS

2 cups fresh kale leaves, roughly torn

2 teaspoons olive oil

Apple cider vinegar, for drizzling

Salt to taste

1 teaspoon Parmesan cheese powder (optional)

METHOD

- Preheat the oven to 150⁰C/300⁰F/Gas Mark 2.
- Place kale leaves on a baking tray. Drizzle some olive oil and vinegar on top and mix gently. Place the baking tray in the preheated oven and cook for five or ten minutes.
- Remove from the oven and sprinkle salt and Parmesan on the crisp kale.
- Serve immediately.

Diet Plans: A B C

Portion: ½-1 cup

Ragi Idli

INGREDIENTS

1 cup finger millet (ragi) flour

½ cup skinless split black gram (dhuli urad dal), soaked for 4 hours and drained

1 cup thick semolina (idli rawa), soaked

1 teaspoon oil + for greasing

1 teaspoon mustard seeds

10-12 curry leaves

1 teaspoon finely chopped green chillies

Salt to taste

A pinch of baking soda (meetha soda)

METHOD

- Grind the black gram with a little water into a smooth paste.
- Drain the semolina and place in a bowl. Add the black gram paste and mix well. Add the millet flour and mix well. Cover the bowl and leave it in a warm place to ferment overnight or for eight hours.
- Heat oil in a non-stick pan; add the mustard seeds and curry leaves and sauté for one minute. Add the green chillies and sauté for half minute. Add the sizzling spices to the fermented batter along with salt and baking soda and mix well.
- Heat sufficient water in a steamer. Grease idli moulds very lightly with oil.
- Pour a ladleful of batter into each mould, place in the steamer, cover and steam for twelve to thirteen minutes.
- Remove the idli from the moulds and serve hot with chutney.

Diet Plans: A B

Portion: 2-3 idli

Spicy Moong Dal Dhokla

INGREDIENTS

1 cup skinless split green gram (dhuli moong dal), soaked for 2 hours

2-3 green chillies, chopped

2 tablespoons chopped fresh fenugreek leaves

2 teaspoons gram flour

2 pinches of asafoetida (hing)

¼ teaspoon fruit salt

2 pinches of sugar

2 teaspoons oil + for greasing

Salt to taste

½ teaspoon mustard seeds

10-12 curry leaves

METHOD

- Blend the soaked green gram in a blender with the green chillies and a little water. Transfer into a bowl.
- Add the fresh fenugreek, gram flour, a pinch of asafoetida, fruit salt, sugar, one teaspoon oil and salt; mix well to make a thick batter.
- Pour the batter into a greased thali and steam in a steamer for about twenty minutes. Remove, cool slightly and cut into squares.
- Heat the remaining oil in a small non-stick pan. Add the mustard seeds, curry leaves, and the remaining asafoetida. Mix and pour over the dhokla.
- Serve hot with Green Chutney (page 307).

Diet Plans: A B C
Portion: 3 pieces

Power Idli

INGREDIENTS

1 cup split skinless black gram, soaked for 2 hours

1 cup split skinless green gram, soaked for 2 hours

3-4 green chillies

1 inch ginger

¼ teaspoon asafoetida

½ teaspoon cumin seeds

¼ teaspoon turmeric powder

Salt to taste

METHOD

- Drain and grind black and green gram until soft and fluffy. Transfer to a deep pan. Cover and leave to ferment overnight or for at least six hours.
- Grind green chillies and ginger to a fine paste, add to the fermented batter and mix well.
- Add asafoetida, cumin seeds, turmeric powder and salt, and stir to mix.
- Heat sufficient water in a steamer. Lightly grease idli moulds. Fill the moulds halfway with the batter, and steam for ten minutes or until set.
- Serve hot with a chutney of your choice.

Diet Plans: A B C
Portion: 3 idli

Ragi Dosa

INGREDIENTS

1 cup finger millet (ragi) flour

¼ cup rice flour

3 tablespoons skinless split black gram (urad dal) flour

2 dried red chillies

½ teaspoon coriander seeds

½ teaspoon fenugreek seeds (methi dana)

310 grams low-fat yogurt

Salt to taste

4 teaspoons oil

METHOD

- Combine the finger millet flour, rice flour and black gram flour in a bowl.
- Grind together the chillies, coriander seeds and fenugreek seeds with a little water to a paste. Mix the yogurt with one cup of water.
- Combine the spice paste and flour mixture. Add the salt, followed by the yogurt-water mixture. Mix well to make a batter of pouring consistency. Leave the batter to rest for three to four hours.
- Heat a non-stick dosa tawa and grease it with a little oil. Sprinkle some water and then wipe the tawa clean with a piece of muslin. This is to prepare the tawa as well as grease it lightly.
- Stir the batter and pour a ladleful on the tawa and spread into a thin, even layer. Cook until crisp and light brown. Remove to a plate. Make the rest of the dosai in the same way. Serve hot.

Diet Plans: A B

Portion: 2 dosai

Soya Shaami Kabab

INGREDIENTS

1¼ cups soya nuggets (wadi)

4 cloves

1 inch cinnamon

1 bay leaf

3 teaspoons oil

1 inch ginger, grated

5 garlic cloves, chopped

4 dried red chillies, broken into 2 pieces

2 green chillies, chopped

½ cup split Bengal gram (chana dal)

1 teaspoon finely crushed dried pomegranate seeds (anardana)

Salt to taste

1 cup breadcrumbs

METHOD

- Soak soya nuggets in hot water for about twenty minutes. Squeeze out excess water.
- Tie the cloves, cinnamon and bay leaf in a piece of muslin to make a small potli.
- Heat one teaspoon of oil in a non-stick pan; add the potli and stir-fry for about two minutes.
- Add the ginger, garlic, red chillies and green chillies and continue to cook for another couple of minutes.

- Add the soya nuggets and Bengal gram and stir for five minutes. Add one cup of water, mix well and lower heat.
- Cook until the gram is cooked and liquid dries completely. Cool the mixture thoroughly, discard the potli, and grind the mixture to a fine paste.
- Add the crushed pomegranate seeds, salt and breadcrumbs and knead into a stiff dough.
- Divide the mixture into eight equal portions. Shape each portion into a round patty (tikki).
- Preheat the air fryer to 180°C. Place the kababs in the fryer basket and cook for ten to fifteen minutes, or according to the manufacturer's instructions. Alternatively, shallow-fry kababs on a lightly greased non-stick tawa or frying pan.
- Serve immediately with a spicy sauce.

Diet Plan: A
Portion: 2 kababs

Mahi Tikka Lehsuni

INGREDIENTS

500 grams boneless white fish, cut into 1½-inch cubes

First marinade

2 teaspoons lemon juice

1 teaspoon garlic paste

1 tablespoon green chilli paste

1 teaspoon black pepper powder

Salt to taste

Second marinade

2 teaspoons oil

3-4 garlic cloves, chopped

½ teaspoon carom seeds (ajwain)

2 tablespoons gram flour (besan)

1 cup low-fat yogurt

¼ teaspoon turmeric powder

½ teaspoon garam masala powder

2 tablespoons chopped fresh coriander

METHOD

- Mix together all the ingredients for the first marinade in a bowl; add the fish, mix and leave to marinate for half an hour.
- For the second marinade, heat the oil in a non-stick pan. Add the garlic, carom seeds and gram flour and sauté until fragrant. Transfer to a bowl and set aside to cool.
- Add the yogurt, turmeric powder, garam masala powder and chopped coriander to the cooled gram flour mixture and mix. Marinate the fish in the second marinade for about one hour.
- Preheat the oven to 200°C/400°F/Gas Mark 6.
- Thread the fish cubes onto skewers and cook in the preheated oven for three to four minutes. Turn the skewers and cook for another five to six minutes, or until the fish is cooked through. Serve hot.

Diet Plans: A C

Portion: 6-8 cubes of fish

Air-Fried Spicy Fish Cakes

INGREDIENTS

400 grams fish fillets, skinned and cut into chunks

3 tablespoons ready-made Thai red curry paste

2 tablespoons fish sauce

2 tablespoons rice flour

Salt to taste

8 kaffir lime leaves, finely shredded

METHOD

- Process the fish chunks and red curry paste in a food processor or blender to a paste. Alternatively, pound the fish and red curry paste with a mortar and pestle.
- Transfer the mixture to a bowl; add the fish sauce, rice flour and salt and knead into a stiff dough. Add the lime leaves and knead again.
- Divide the mixture into eight equal portions and shape into balls. Flatten each ball with moistened hands into a half-inch thick round cake or patty (tikki).
- Preheat the air fryer to 180°C. Place the cakes in the basket and cook for ten to twelve minutes.
- Alternatively, heat two teaspoons oil in a non-stick frying pan and fry the fish cakes, a few at a time, for four or five minutes on each side, or until cooked and golden.
- Serve hot with sauce.

Diet Plans: A C

Portion: 2 cakes

Chicken Frankies

INGREDIENTS

400 grams boneless chicken, cut into ½-inch pieces

1½ cups whole-wheat flour (atta)

Salt to taste

2 teaspoons oil

2 medium onions, roughly chopped

2 medium tomatoes, chopped

2 teaspoons ginger paste

2 teaspoons garlic paste

2 teaspoons Kashmiri red chilli powder

½ teaspoon turmeric powder

2 teaspoons coriander powder

2 tablespoons lemon juice

4 egg whites

To serve

2 medium onions, sliced

8 teaspoons Green Chutney (page 307)

METHOD

- Mix flour and salt, add sufficient water and knead to make a firm dough.
- Cover and leave to rest for about fifteen minutes.
- Divide into eight equal balls and roll out into roti.
- Cook them lightly on a non-stick tawa and set aside.

- Heat two teaspoons of oil in a non-stick pan; add onions, tomatoes, ginger paste, garlic paste, chicken, salt, chilli powder, turmeric powder and coriander powder, and stir on high heat until the chicken is cooked. Stir in the lemon juice.
- Beat egg whites with salt in a bowl.
- Heat a non-stick tawa and place a roti on it. Spread a little beaten egg white on the roti. Turn it over and spread a little egg white on the other side as well. Flip over and cook until the egg has just set–do not overcook.
- Place a little chicken mixture on one side of the roti. Sprinkle sliced onion over the chicken. Spread some green chutney on top and roll up the roti pressing it firmly to enclose the filling.
- Wrap in greaseproof paper or aluminium foil and serve immediately.

Diet Plan: A

Portion: 1 frankie

Chicken Tikka Chaat

INGREDIENTS

2 skinless boneless chicken breasts (approx. 300 grams), skinned and cubed

1 teaspoon Kashmiri red chilli powder

1 teaspoon ginger paste

1 teaspoon garlic paste

1 cup drained (hung) skimmed milk yogurt

Salt to taste

½ teaspoon garam masala powder

2 tablespoons lemon juice

3 teaspoons olive oil

1 small green capsicum, diced

1 small red capsicum, diced

1 small yellow capsicum, diced

1 medium onion, sliced

2 green chillies, chopped

1 teaspoon chaat masala

2 tablespoons chopped fresh coriander

½ small unripe mango, chopped (optional)

METHOD

- Combine the chilli powder, ginger and garlic pastes, yogurt, salt, garam masala powder, one tablespoon lemon juice and two teaspoons of olive oil in a bowl.

- Add the chicken and mix well. Set aside to marinate for three to four hours, preferably in the refrigerator.
- Preheat an oven to 200°C/400°F/Gas Mark 6. Alternatively, preheat a tandoor.
- Thread the chicken pieces onto skewers and cook in the preheated oven, or a moderately hot tandoor, for ten to twelve minutes, or until almost cooked. Baste the chicken with the remaining oil and cook for another four minutes. Set aside to cool. Remove the chicken from the skewers.
- Combine the chicken tikka with the capsicums, onion, chillies, chaat masala, half the chopped coriander, the remaining lemon juice and the mango, and toss well to mix.
- Transfer to a serving dish and serve, garnished with the remaining chopped coriander.

Diet Plans: A C

Portion: 6-8 pieces chicken

Yakitori Chicken with Spring Onions

INGREDIENTS

400 grams boneless chicken thigh or breast pieces, cut into 1½-inch cubes

4 spring onions, halved

1 large red capsicum, cut into 1-inch pieces

4 button mushrooms, halved

8 fresh shiitake mushrooms, halved

2 teaspoons oil

8 satay sticks, soaked in warm water

Sauce

2 tablespoons white wine vinegar diluted with 2 tablespoons water

2 tablespoons soy sauce (preferably Japanese)

2 teaspoons sugar or equivalent sugar substitute

½ teaspoon black pepper powder

METHOD

- To make the sauce, pour white wine vinegar into a small non-stick pan; add the soy sauce and sugar and bring the mixture to a boil.
- Add pepper powder and mix.

- Lower the heat and simmer, uncovered, over medium heat until the sauce reduces to one-third. Cool.
- Thread the ingredients onto satay sticks in the following order: a spring onion half, two chicken cubes, a piece of red capsicum, half a button mushroom, a shiitake mushroom, two more chicken cubes and finally a piece of red capsicum.
- Leave a little space between each ingredient to allow even cooking.
- Heat oil on a non-stick tawa. Place four satay sticks at a time on it and cook, turning and brushing with the sauce occasionally, until brown and cooked through.
- Serve the yakitori sprinkled with remaining sauce.

Diet Plans: A C

Portion: 2 skewers (8 chicken cubes)

Carrot and Onion Florentine

INGREDIENTS

3-4 medium carrots, cut into ½-inch cubes

2 medium onions, thinly sliced

2 medium bundles (250 grams each) spinach, finely chopped

1 teaspoon oil

6-7 garlic cloves, crushed

Salt to taste

White pepper powder to taste

2 cups skimmed milk

100 grams broad beans (papdi), cut into ½-inch pieces

2 tablespoons cornflour, mixed with ¼ cup water

¼ teaspoon dried mixed herbs

¼ cup fresh whole-wheat breadcrumbs

METHOD

- Preheat the oven to 180°C/350°F/Gas Mark 4.
- Heat oil in a non-stick pan; add half the garlic, stir briefly and add the spinach. Sauté over high heat for four to five minutes, or until the spinach is cooked completely.
- Add salt and white pepper powder to taste, stir well and remove from heat.
- Heat the skimmed milk in a non-stick pan and bring to a boil.

- Add the remaining garlic, the carrots, broad beans and onions. Cover and simmer for three to four minutes, stirring frequently. Add salt and white pepper powder to taste.
- Gradually add the cornflour mixture, stirring continuously, until the mixture thickens to the consistency of a moderately thick sauce. Add the mixed herbs, stir well, remove from heat and keep warm.
- Spread the cooked spinach in an ovenproof glass dish. Pour the cooked vegetables with the sauce over the spinach and level the top with a spatula.
- Sprinkle the breadcrumbs on top and bake in the preheated oven for ten minutes. Serve hot.

Diet Plans: A B C

Portion: 1 bowl (1½ katori)

Chinese Stir-Fried Vegetables

INGREDIENTS

100 grams bean curd (tofu), cut into 8-10 pieces

½ medium broccoli, separated into small florets

1 medium carrot, halved and sliced diagonally into 1-inch pieces

4-6 small pieces baby corn, sliced diagonally into 1-inch pieces

4-6 button mushrooms, quartered

4-6 French beans, sliced diagonally into 1-inch pieces

1 medium green capsicum, sliced diagonally into 1-inch pieces

¼ small Chinese cabbage, sliced diagonally into 1-inch pieces

10-12 spinach leaves, torn into 2 pieces

Salt to taste

1 tablespoon cornflour

2 teaspoons oil

6-8 garlic cloves, crushed

2 spring onions with greens, sliced

METHOD

- Soak the bean curd in hot, salted water for five minutes. Drain and set aside.
- Soak the broccoli florets in warm salted water for fifteen minutes. Drain and set aside.
- Mix cornflour in one cup of water.
- Heat oil in a non-stick wok; add garlic and sliced spring onion bulbs, reserving the greens for garnish, and stir-fry for half a minute.

1 teaspoon sugar or equivalent sugar substitute
1 tablespoons light soy sauce
½ teaspoon white pepper powder
1 teaspoon toasted sesame seeds (til)

- Add carrot, baby corn, mushrooms and broccoli and continue to stir-fry.
- Add French beans, capsicum and Chinese cabbage and cook for two to three minutes.
- Stir in one cup of water and simmer for a couple of minutes. Add salt, sugar, soy sauce and white pepper powder.
- Add spinach leaves and bean curd. Stir in the cornflour mixture, and cook, stirring, until the sauce thickens and coats all the vegetables.
- Sprinkle with toasted sesame seeds and serve hot, garnished with the reserved spring onion greens.

Diet Plans: A B C

Portion: 1 bowl (1½ katori)

Hunan-Style Hot and Sour Vegetables

INGREDIENTS

¼ small cauliflower, separated into small florets

1 medium carrot, sliced thinly

1 medium zucchini, sliced thinly

2 tablespoons black bean sauce

1 inch ginger, chopped

4-5 garlic cloves, chopped

¼ teaspoon red chilli flakes

2 cups Vegetable Stock (page 307)

1 tablespoon soy sauce

1 tablespoon white vinegar

¼ teaspoon sugar

2 teaspoons oil

2 tablespoons cornflour

3-4 spring onions green leaves, sliced diagonally

METHOD

- Blanch cauliflower in boiling water for two minutes. Refresh in chilled water. Drain and set aside. Mix black bean sauce, ginger, garlic and red chilli flakes in a bowl and set aside.
- Blend together vegetable stock, soy sauce, white vinegar and sugar in another bowl and set aside.
- Heat oil in a non-stick wok or pan; add black bean sauce mixture and stir-fry for half a minute. Add the blanched cauliflower along with carrot and zucchini and toss for two to three minutes. Add stock mixture and stir well. Bring to a boil, reduce heat, cover and cook for one minute taking care that the vegetables remain crisp.
- Mix the cornflour in one-fourth cup of water and add to the pan. Stir and cook for a minute and remove from heat.Garnish with spring onion greens and serve hot.

Diet Plans: A B C

Portion: 1 bowl (1½ katori)

Spinach with Green Peas

INGREDIENTS

2 medium bunches (500 grams) spinach, cleaned

¼ cup frozen green peas

2 green chillies

2 small onions, roughly chopped

1 inch ginger

4 garlic cloves

1 teaspoon garam masala powder

Salt to taste

1 teaspoon coriander powder

1 teaspoon cumin powder

4 tablespoons low-fat milk

METHOD

- Blend together the green chillies, onions, ginger and garlic into a smooth paste.
- Blanch the spinach in one cup of water for a minute. Drain and blend into a smooth purée.
- Heat a non-stick pan; add the spice paste and spinach purée and cook, stirring, for three to four minutes. Add the green peas, garam masala powder, salt, coriander powder, cumin powder and milk, and mix well. Cook for four to five minutes. Serve hot.

Recipe courtesy Dr Sarita Davare

Diet Plans: A B C

Portion: 1 bowl (1½ katori)

Main Dishes - Vegetables

Achari Baingan

INGREDIENTS

8-10 small brinjals (baingan) with stems, slit into 4

2 teaspoons oil

½ teaspoon mustard seeds

1 teaspoon fennel seeds

½ teaspoon onion seeds

¼ teaspoon turmeric powder

2 teaspoons coriander powder

1 teaspoon red chilli powder

2 teaspoons ginger-garlic paste

1 medium onion, chopped

½ cup tomato purée

Salt to taste

2-3 green chillies, chopped

1 tablespoon chopped fresh coriander

METHOD

- Heat the oil in a non-stick pan. Add the mustard seeds, fennel seeds and onion seeds.
- When the mustard seeds start to splutter, add the turmeric powder, coriander powder and chilli powder and sauté for a few seconds.
- Add the ginger-garlic paste and sauté until the raw flavour disappears. Add the onion and sauté until golden.
- Add the tomato purée and sauté until the oil separates.
- Add the salt, green chillies, brinjals and one cup of water. Cook, covered, on low heat for ten minutes.
- Serve hot, garnished with chopped coriander.

Diet Plans: A B C

Portion: 1 bowl (1½ katori)

Cauliflower Santa Fé

INGREDIENTS

1 medium cauliflower, separated into small florets

Salt to taste

1 teaspoon oil

2 medium onions, chopped

5 garlic cloves, chopped

4-5 medium tomatoes, puréed

1 dried red chilli, crushed coarsely

¾ cup cream-style sweet corn

3-4 pickled jalapeño peppers, roughly chopped

½ cup whole-wheat breadcrumbs

METHOD

- Soak the cauliflower florets in salted water for fifteen minutes. Drain and refresh in plain water. Drain again and set aside.
- Preheat the oven to 180ºC/350ºF/Gas Mark 4.
- Heat oil in a non-stick pan; add onion and sauté until soft and translucent. Add garlic and sauté for a few seconds. Add cauliflower and half a cup of water. Cover and cook on medium heat for ten minutes, stirring occasionally. Add tomato purée, crushed red chilli and salt.
- Cover and cook on medium heat for five to six minutes, stirring occasionally. Stir in the cream-style corn and pickled jalapeños.
- Remove from heat, pour into an ovenproof dish and sprinkle breadcrumbs on top. Place in the preheated oven and bake for ten minutes. Serve hot.

Chef's Tip

Jalapeño (pronounced hala-penyo) peppers can be replaced with thick green chillies that are not too hot.

Diet Plans: A B C

Portion: 1 bowl (1½ katori)

Masaledaar Tofu Bhurji

INGREDIENTS

300 grams bean curd (tofu)

1½ teaspoons olive oil or rice bran oil

1 teaspoon cumin seeds

2 medium onions, chopped

1 inch ginger, chopped

2 green chillies, chopped

½ teaspoon turmeric powder

1teaspoon red chilli powder

1 tablespoon coriander powder

1 teaspoon cumin powder

2 medium tomatoes, chopped

2 medium green capsicums, seeded and chopped

Salt to taste

¼ cup chopped fresh coriander

METHOD

- Drain the bean curd and crumble it into small pieces.
- Heat the oil in a non-stick pan and add the cumin seeds. When they begin to change colour, add the onion, ginger and green chillies. Stir-fry until onion becomes translucent.
- Mix the turmeric powder, chilli powder, coriander powder and cumin powder in half a cup of water and add the mixture to the pan. Cook on medium heat for half a minute, stirring continuously. Add the tomatoes and cook on high heat for two minutes, stirring continuously. Stir in the crumbled bean curd, capsicum and salt to taste. Mix well. Reduce heat and cook for two to three minutes, tossing frequently to prevent scorching.
- Sprinkle the chopped coriander on top and serve.

Diet Plans: A B C

Portion: 1 bowl (1½ katori)

Masaledar Karele

INGREDIENTS

12 medium-sized bitter gourds (karele)

Salt to taste

2 teaspoons coriander powder

2 teaspoons cumin powder

¾ teaspoon turmeric powder

1½ tablespoons dried mango powder (amchur)

¾ tablespoon red chilli powder

½ tablespoon garam masala powder

3½ tablespoons fennel seeds (saunf)

3 teaspoons oil

2 large onions, finely chopped

1 teaspoon sugar or equivalent sugar substitute

METHOD

- Scrape the bitter gourds. Slit and remove seeds. Apply salt and set aside for half an hour. Squeeze lightly and wash under running water. Wipe dry and set aside.
- Dry-roast all the spice powders one by one on low heat until fragrant. Dry-roast the fennel seeds and grind coarsely. Mix together with the roasted spice powders.
- Heat one and a half teaspoons of oil in a non-stick pan; add the onions and sauté until golden. Remove from heat and add the spice powder mixture, salt and sugar. Mix well.
- Fill the bitter gourds with the onion and spice mixture.
- Heat the remaining oil in a wide non-stick pan. Arrange the bitter gourds in the pan. Cover with a tight lid and cook over low heat until tender. Remove the lid and sauté the gourds until lightly browned. Serve hot.

Diet Plans: A B C

Portion: 2-3 stuffed bitter gourds

Santung Garden Vegetables

INGREDIENTS

3-4 baby carrots, halved lengthways

2 celery stalks, sliced

2 leeks, sliced

8-10 snow peas or flat beans, halved

6-8 pieces baby corn, halved lengthways

4 medium zucchini, cut into thin round slices

100 grams bean curd (tofu), cut into 1-inch pieces

2 slices pineapple, cut into 1-inch pieces

1 tablespoon cornflour

2 teaspoons oil

1 star anise (chakri phool/badiyan)

1 teaspoon Chinese Five-Spice Powder (see Chef's Tip below)

2 tablespoons lemon juice

1 teaspoon honey

Salt to taste

¼ teaspoon black pepper powder

½ teaspoon grated lemon rind

A few celery leaves

METHOD

- Mix the cornflour with one-fourth cup of water. Set aside.
- Heat the oil in a non-stick wok.
- Add the star anise, baby carrots, celery stems, leeks, snow peas and baby corn.
- Stir-fry for about three to four minutes on high heat.

- Add the five-spice powder and stir to mix. Add zucchini, bean curd and pineapple and stir gently.
- Add half a cup of hot water and bring to a boil. Stir in cornflour mixture and cook for half a minute on high heat, stirring continuously.
- Stir in lemon juice and honey. Add salt and pepper powder and mix.
- Serve hot, garnished with lemon rind and celery leaves.

Chef's Tip

Chinese five-spice powder can be made at home by grinding together equal quantities of star anise, cinnamon, fennel seeds, cloves and Sichuan peppers.

Diet Plans: A B C

Portion: 1 bowl (1½ katori)

Mushroom Balchão

INGREDIENTS

600 grams fresh button mushrooms, quartered

10-12 dried red chillies

8-10 garlic cloves

1 inch ginger

1 teaspoon cumin seeds

7-8 cloves

1 teaspoon mustard seeds

1 inch cinnamon

Salt to taste

½ cup malt vinegar

2 teaspoons olive oil or rice bran oil

2 medium onions, chopped

2 medium tomatoes, chopped

¾ cup tomato purée

2 teaspoons sugar

METHOD

- Grind the red chillies, garlic, ginger, cumin seeds, cloves, mustard seeds, cinnamon and salt with one-fourth cup of malt vinegar to a fine paste.
- Heat the oil in a non-stick kadai; add the onions and sauté until light brown. Add the tomatoes, mix well and cook for five minutes, stirring continuously.
- Add the mushrooms, tomato purée and the ground spice paste and cook for three or four minutes. Add the sugar, more salt if necessary and mix well.
- Stir in the remaining malt vinegar and cook for five to seven minutes. Serve hot.

Diet Plans: A B C

Portion: 1 bowl (1½ katori)

Broccoli in Orange Sauce

INGREDIENTS

2 medium heads broccoli

2 large oranges

2 tablespoons cornflour

2 teaspoons light soy sauce

1 teaspoon honey

2 teaspoons oil

2 medium carrots, thinly sliced

1 inch ginger, thinly sliced

4-6 garlic cloves, thinly sliced

Salt to taste

Black pepper powder to taste

METHOD

- Separate the broccoli into small florets; peel the stem and cut into thin slices.
- Squeeze the oranges and mix the juice with the cornflour, soy sauce, honey and half a cup of water. Cut a small piece of orange peel into thin strips and soak them in cold water.
- Heat the oil in a non-stick pan; add the broccoli stems and carrots and sauté for about two minutes.
- Add ginger, garlic and broccoli florets and sauté for another two minutes. Sprinkle a little water and cook for a few more minutes.
- Stir in the orange juice mixture and cook on high heat for about a minute, stirring continuously. Do not overcook. Add salt and pepper powder. Drain the orange peel and stir into the pan before serving.

Diet Plans: A B C

Portion: 1 bowl (1½ katori)

Main Dishes - Vegetables

Sing nu Shaak

INGREDIENTS

8 drumsticks (saijan/sing)

1 cup gram flour (besan)

Salt to taste

1½ teaspoons coriander-cumin powder

½ teaspoon turmeric powder

1 teaspoon red chilli powder

3 tablespoons Tamarind Pulp (page 307)

2 teaspoons grated jaggery

1 teaspoon garam masala powder

METHOD

- Cut the drumsticks into one-and-a-half-inch pieces, removing strings in the process. Boil in sufficient water until done.
- Roast the gram flour in a non-stick pan on low heat until fragrant. Transfer to a bowl. Add salt, coriander-cumin powder, turmeric powder, chilli powder, tamarind pulp, jaggery, garam masala powder and a little water and mix to a smooth paste. Add two cups of water and mix well.
- Heat a non-stick pan; add the gram flour mixture and cook for two to three minutes. Add the drumsticks, add more water if necessary, and cook for five to ten minutes on medium heat. Serve hot.

Diet Plans: A B C

Portion: 1 bowl (1½ katori)

Soya Keema

INGREDIENTS

1 cup soya granules

1½ cups skimmed milk

2 medium onions, finely chopped

8 garlic cloves, finely chopped

1 inch ginger, grated

2 green chillies, chopped

1 teaspoon coriander powder

1 teaspoon cumin powder

¾ teaspoon red chilli powder

1 cup shelled green peas

4 tablespoons chopped fresh coriander

Salt to taste

1 teaspoon garam masala powder

1 tablespoon lemon juice

METHOD

- Soak the soya granules in the milk for an hour.
- Heat a non-stick pan; add chopped onions and cook, stirring, until lightly browned. Add garlic and cook for a minute, stirring continuously.
- Add grated ginger, green chillies, coriander powder, cumin powder, chilli powder and two tablespoons of water. Stir and cook for two minutes.
- Add green peas and one-fourth cup of water and mix well. Cover and cook until peas are nearly tender.
- Add soya granules along with the milk and cook until almost dry. Add chopped coriander, salt, garam masala powder and lemon juice and mix well. Serve hot.

Diet Plans: A B C

Portion: 1 bowl (1½ katori)

Green Tomato Curry

INGREDIENTS

8 medium green tomatoes, seeded and minced

2 teaspoons split green gram (chilkewali moong dal), soaked

2 green chillies, chopped

2 medium onions, chopped

A pinch of turmeric powder

½ teaspoon red chilli powder

½ teaspoon coriander-cumin powder

Salt to taste

2 teaspoons finely chopped fresh coriander

METHOD

- Heat a non-stick pan; add the green chillies, onions and green gram and cook, stirring continuously, for three to four minutes.
- Add the green tomatoes, turmeric powder, chilli powder, coriander-cumin powder and salt, mix well and cook until tomatoes are soft.
- Add the chopped coriander and mix well. Add one cup of water, mix well and cook for five to six minutes.
- Serve hot.

Recipe courtesy Dr Sarita Davare

Diet Plans: A B C

Portion: 1 bowl (1½ katori)

Stuffed Lady's Fingers

INGREDIENTS

20 tender lady's fingers, slit

4 teaspoons oil

4 teaspoons Kitchen King masala

¼ teaspoon turmeric powder

¼ teaspoon red chilli powder

¼ teaspoon coriander-cumin powder

¼ teaspoon chaat masala

¼ teaspoon dried mango powder (amchur)

¼ teaspoon salt

METHOD

- Lightly rub the lady's fingers with oil.
- To make the masala mixture, combine the Kitchen King masala, turmeric powder, chilli powder, coriander-cumin powder, chaat masala, dried mango powder and salt in a bowl and mix well.
- Stuff the lady's fingers with the prepared masala mixture.
- Heat a non-stick frying pan; add the stuffed lady's fingers and cook, turning the vegetables occasionally, for five to seven minutes.
- Serve hot.

Recipe courtesy Dr Sarita Davare

Diet Plans: A B C

Portion: 1 bowl (1½ katori)

Main Dishes - Vegetables

Soya Nuggets with Mushrooms

INGREDIENTS

20 soya bean chunks or nuggets

20 button mushrooms, halved and washed

4 teaspoons ginger-garlic paste

2 medium onions, chopped

Pulp of 2 medium tomatoes

¼ teaspoon turmeric powder

1 teaspoon red chilli powder

1 teaspoon coriander-cumin powder

1 teaspoon salt

METHOD

- Soak the soya bean chunks in three cups of hot water for twenty minutes. Drain and set aside.
- Heat a non-stick pan; add the ginger-garlic paste, onion and tomato pulp and cook, stirring continuously, for three to four minutes.
- Add the turmeric powder, chilli powder, coriander-cumin powder, salt and stir to mix.
- Add the drained soya bean chunks and mushrooms and mix well. Add three to four tablespoons of water, mix, cover and cook for three to four minutes.
- Serve hot.

Recipe courtesy Dr Sarita Davare

Diet Plans: A B C

Portion: 1 bowl (1½ katori)

Bhapa Ilish

INGREDIENTS

500 grams hilsa (ilish), seer fish (surmai) or Indian salmon (rawas)

Salt to taste

1 teaspoon turmeric powder

1 teaspoon yellow mustard seeds

1 teaspoon black mustard seeds

2-3 green chillies

1 inch ginger, sliced

2 teaspoons mustard oil

METHOD

- Wash the fish well and clean it. Cut into darnes (slices across the bone). Sprinkle salt and half the turmeric powder and set aside for ten to fifteen minutes.
- Grind together yellow mustard seeds, black mustard seeds, green chillies, ginger, remaining turmeric powder and salt to a fine paste.
- Place the fish in a non-stick pan that will fit in a pressure cooker. Spread the paste liberally all over the fish. Drizzle mustard oil on top. Pour three cups of water into a pressure cooker and place a ring or upturned bowl in it. Place the pan with the fish on the ring.
- Cover with the lid and steam without the weight for eight to ten minutes. Serve hot.

Diet Plans: A C

Portion: 2 slices fish

Baked Fish in Red Masala

INGREDIENTS

2 whole (600 grams each) pomfrets

Salt to taste

2 tablespoons lemon juice

¼ teaspoon turmeric powder

2-3 banana leaves

2 lemons, cut into wedges

2 medium onions, cut into rings

Masala paste

6 dried red chillies

2 teaspoons coriander seeds

2 teaspoons cumin seeds

5-6 black peppercorns

4-5 cloves

½ inch cinnamon

8 garlic cloves

1 inch ginger

1 medium tomato, roughly chopped

2 tablespoons vinegar

½ teaspoon sugar

Salt to taste

METHOD

- Wash, clean and pat the fish dry. Make diagonal slits on both sides of the fish using a sharp knife.
- Rub salt, lemon juice and turmeric powder on the inside and outside of the fish.
- Marinate for half an hour, preferably in the refrigerator.

- Preheat the oven to 200°C/400°F/Gas Mark 6.
- Combine all the ingredients for the masala paste and grind to a smooth paste, using a little water if required.
- Apply the paste on both the sides of the fish and marinate for fifteen minutes, preferably in the refrigerator.
- Wrap the fish in banana leaves and place them on a baking tray. Place in the preheated oven and bake for ten to fifteen minutes.
- Serve hot with lemon wedges and onion rings.

Diet Plans: A C

Portion: ½ pomfret

Five-Spice Fish

INGREDIENTS

400 grams bonless seer fish (surmai) or Indian salmon (rawas) fillets, cut into 1½-inch pieces

1 star anise (chakhri phool/badiyan)

½ tablespoon fennel seeds (saunf)

1 inch cinnamon

5 black peppercorns

½ inch ginger, crushed

½ tablespoon cornflour

½ spring onion with greens

2 cups Fish Stock (page 307)

2 teaspoons dark soy sauce

½ teaspoon sugar

2 teaspoons sesame (til) oil

1 green chilli, slit

1-inch piece of leek, chopped

½ celery stalk, chopped

METHOD

- Tie star anise, fennel seeds, cinnamon, black peppercorns and ginger in a piece of muslin to make a spice bundle (potli).
- Mix cornflour and four tablespoons of water and set aside.
- Slice the spring onion bulb and reserve the greens for garnish.

- Pour the fish stock into a deep non-stick pan. Add soy sauce, sugar and the spice bundle.
- Stir, and bring the mixture to a boil. Simmer for ten minutes. Take the pan off the heat and remove the spice bundle.
- Heat the sesame oil in a non-stick wok; add the green chillies, spring onion, leek and celery and stir-fry for two minutes.
- Add the fish and toss gently over high heat for about two to three minutes. Add the flavoured fish stock and bring to a boil.
- Add the cornflour mixture and cook, stirring continuously, until the sauce thickens.
- Serve hot, garnished with spring onion greens.

Diet Plans: A C

Portion: 1 cup (1 katori) with 6-8 pieces fish

Grilled Fish with Salsa

INGREDIENTS

400 grams seer fish (surmai), cut into 8 darnes (slices on the bone)

Salt to taste

3 tablespoons lemon juice

2 tablespoons malt vinegar

2 tablespoons English mustard paste

1 tablespoon ginger-garlic paste

1 tablespoon red chilli sauce

16 cloves

Salsa

½ cup corn kernels

10-12 fresh basil leaves (tulsi), wiped dry

1 large onion, roasted and finely chopped

4-5 garlic cloves, roasted and finely chopped

2 medium tomatoes, chopped

2 pineapple slices, chopped

1 jalapeño pepper, finely chopped (see Chef's Tip on page 231)

Salt to taste

1 tablespoon lemon juice

2 tablespoons finely chopped fresh coriander

METHOD

- Marinate the fish slices in a mixture of salt, lemon juice, malt vinegar, English mustard paste, ginger-garlic paste and red chilli sauce for half an hour.
- Preheat a non-stick grill.
- Stud marinated fish slices with cloves; place them on the hot grill and cook, turning once, for eight to ten minutes or until fish flakes easily with a fork. Do not overcook the fish. Remove the cloves.

- To make salsa, cook corn kernels with half a cup of water in a microwave-safe bowl on HIGH for one minute. Drain.
- Tear basil leaves, reserving a few whole leaves for garnish.
- Mix together corn, onion, garlic, tomatoes, pineapple, jalapeño pepper, salt, basil leaves, lemon juice and chopped coriander.
- Place salsa on a platter and arrange grilled fish on the salsa; garnish with reserved basil leaves and serve.

Diet Plans: A C

Portion: 2 slices fish with 1 cup (1 katori) salsa

Greek-Style Yogurt Chicken

INGREDIENTS

4 (600 grams) skinless, boneless chicken breasts

½ cup skimmed milk yogurt

2 tablespoons lemon juice

8-10 garlic cloves, ground to a paste

1½ teaspoons olive oil

½ teaspoon paprika

½ teaspoon crushed black peppercorns

Salt to taste

1 tablespoon chopped fresh parsley

2 tablespoons chopped fresh coriander

10-12 fresh mint leaves, chopped

1 teaspoon oil

6-8 black olives, stoned

METHOD

- Make three slits on each chicken breast.
- Tie the yogurt in a piece of muslin for about ten to fifteen minutes to drain the whey. Transfer the drained yogurt to a bowl.
- Add lemon juice, garlic paste, olive oil, paprika, crushed peppercorns, salt, half each of the parsley, chopped coriander and mint leaves.

- Marinate the chicken in the mixture, preferably in a refrigerator, for one hour.
- Heat a shallow non-stick pan and brush it with the oil.
- Add the chicken breasts and sear on high heat for one minute on each side.
- Reduce heat, cover and cook, turning the pieces occasionally for uniform cooking and browning, for eight to ten minutes, or until completely cooked.
- Add the black olives, stir and transfer to a serving dish.
- Garnish with the remaining parsley, coriander and mint and serve hot.

Chef's Tip

You may substitute paprika with red chilli powder that is not too hot and is bright red in colour e.g. Kashmiri red chilli powder or deghi mirch powder.

Diet Plans: A C
Portion: 1 chicken breast

Handi Murgh

INGREDIENTS

1 medium chicken, skinned and cut into 8 pieces on the bone

1 teaspoon poppy seeds (khus khus)

4-5 green chillies, roughly chopped

½ cup fresh coriander, roughly chopped

¼ cup fresh mint, roughly chopped

2 inches ginger, roughly chopped

10-12 garlic cloves, roughly chopped

1 teaspoon fenugreek seeds (methi dana)

1 teaspoon fennel seeds (saunf)

2 tablespoons coriander seeds

1 teaspoon cumin seeds

¼ cup skimmed milk yogurt

Salt to taste

½ teaspoon turmeric powder

1 teaspoon garam masala powder

2 medium onions, finely grated

2 medium tomatoes, quartered

METHOD

- Soak the poppy seeds in one-fourth cup of warm water for fifteen to twenty minutes.
- Grind the green chillies, chopped coriander, mint, ginger, garlic and soaked poppy seeds to a smooth, fine paste.
- Dry-roast fenugreek seeds, fennel seeds, coriander seeds and cumin seeds lightly on a non-stick tawa and grind to a powder.

- In a bowl, mix together the chicken, green spice paste, freshly ground spice powder, skimmed milk yogurt, salt, turmeric powder and garam masala powder. Marinate for one hour in the refrigerator.
- Place the chicken in a thick-bottomed non-stick handi (a vessel with a narrow mouth); add the onion, tomatoes and half a cup of water and mix well.
- Seal the handi with a tight fitting lid or with whole-wheat (atta) dough. Place the handi on medium heat and cook for eight to ten minutes.
- Reduce heat and place the handi on a hot non-stick tawa and simmer for ten to fifteen minutes. Alternatively, place the handi in an oven preheated to 150-170°C/300-325°F/ Gas Mark 2-3 for fifteen minutes.
- Carefully break open the seal just before serving to retain the flavour and aroma.

Diet Plans: A C

Portion: 1 cup (1 katori) with 2 pieces chicken on the bone

Kung Pao Chicken

INGREDIENTS

400 grams boneless chicken breasts, cut into 1-inch cubes

2 egg whites

6 tablespoons cornflour

1½ tablespoons lemon juice

½ teaspoon white pepper powder

Salt to taste

5 teaspoons oil

5-6 dried red chillies, broken in half

1 inch ginger, finely chopped

4-5 garlic cloves, finely chopped

2 spring onions with greens, finely chopped

2 tablespoons soy sauce

1 teaspoons sugar

3 tablespoons rice wine (optional)

½ cup Chicken Stock (page 307)

1 tablespoon roasted peanuts

1 teaspoon chilli oil

METHOD

- Mix the egg whites, four tablespoons of cornflour, the lemon juice, white pepper, salt and chicken in a bowl.
- Marinate for half an hour preferably in the refrigerator.
- Mix the remaining cornflour in half a cup of water. Set aside.

- Heat three teaspoons oil in a non-stick wok; add the marinated chicken and sauté for three minutes, or until the chicken is light golden brown in colour. Drain on absorbent paper.
- Heat remaining oil in a non-stick wok or a pan; add the red chillies, ginger and garlic and stir-fry for a minute.
- Add the spring onions, reserving the greens for garnishing, and continue to stir-fry for a minute more.
- Add the soy sauce, sugar, rice wine and salt, and mix. Stir in the chicken stock and cook for a few minutes.
- Stir in the cornflour mixture and immediately add the sautéed chicken and peanuts. Stir-fry for two minutes on high heat.
- Drizzle the chilli oil over the chicken and serve hot, garnished with the reserved spring onion greens.

Chef's Tip

You can substitute the peanuts with roasted cashew nuts or almonds.

Diet Plans: A C

Portion: 1 cup (1 katori) with 6-8 pieces chicken

Saagwala Murgh

INGREDIENTS

3 medium bunches (250 grams each) spinach

400 grams boneless chicken, cut into 1½-inch cubes

½ cup skimmed milk yogurt

1 tablespoon ginger-garlic paste

½ teaspoon turmeric powder

2 teaspoons red chilli powder

½ teaspoon coriander powder

1 teaspoon garam masala powder

Salt to taste

3-4 green chillies

2 bay leaves (tej pata)

3 green cardamoms

1 black cardamom

6 cloves

1 inch cinnamon

6-8 black peppercorns

1 teaspoon cumin seeds

6-8 garlic cloves, chopped

3 medium onions, sliced

METHOD

- In a bowl, mix together half the yogurt, the ginger-garlic paste, turmeric powder, one teaspoon of chilli powder, coriander powder, garam masala powder and salt to taste.
- Marinate the chicken in this mixture for about half an hour.
- Blanch the spinach in salted boiling water for one minute. Drain and refresh in cold water.

1 inch ginger, cut into thin strips

½ tablespoon fresh dill leaves (suva), chopped

1 teaspoon dried fenugreek leaves (kasoori methi), roasted and crushed

- Grind spinach and green chillies together to a coarse paste.
- Heat a thick-bottomed non-stick pan and roast bay leaves, green cardamoms, black cardamom, cloves, cinnamon, peppercorns and cumin seeds until fragrant. Add garlic and roast until light brown. Add onions and cook until translucent.
- Add half the ginger strips, remaining chilli powder and marinated chicken.
- Cook on high heat, stirring continuously, for two minutes. Add remaining yogurt, and one cup of water and bring to a boil. Cover and cook for seven to eight minutes.
- Add spinach paste and dill leaves and stir. Adjust seasonings and cook until the chicken is tender and spinach is soft.
- Sprinkle dried fenugreek leaves and serve hot, garnished with remaining ginger strips.

Diet Plans: A C

Portion: 1 cup (1 katori) with 6-8 pieces chicken

Braised Sichuan Chicken

INGREDIENTS

400 grams boneless chicken breast, cut into 1-inch pieces

4-5 dried black mushrooms

1 tablespoon cornflour

1½ teaspoons hot soy bean paste *

1 teaspoon sugar or equivalent sugar substitute

½ teaspoon white pepper powder

1 tablespoon rice wine (optional)

Salt to taste

1 cup Chicken Stock (page 307)

2 teaspoons oil

1 inch ginger, thinly sliced

4-5 dried red chillies, torn in half

2 spring onions, cut into 1-inch long pieces

2 teaspoons chilli oil

* Use a mixture of 1 teaspoon oyster sauce and ½ teaspoon chilli sauce to get an approximate flavor. Reduce the sugar.

METHOD

- Pat the chicken pieces dry thoroughly with a clean kitchen towel.
- Soak the mushrooms in sufficient hot water for fifteen minutes. Drain and cut them into quarters.
- Mix cornflour in half a cup of water.
- In a bowl, combine the soy bean paste, sugar, pepper, rice wine, salt and chicken stock.

- Heat the oil in a wok or pan. Add the ginger and red chillies and stir-fry for half a minute.
- Add the chicken, spring onions and mushrooms, and continue to stir-fry for a couple of minutes more, or until the chicken is cooked.
- Stir in the sauce and spice mixture, and cook on medium heat for a minute. Stir in the cornflour mixture.
- Cook on high heat for half a minute or until the sauce coats the chicken well, stirring continuously.
- Drizzle chilli oil over the chicken and serve hot.

Diet Plans: A C

Portion: 1 cup (1 katori) with 6-8 pieces chicken

Tamatar Murgh Kofta

INGREDIENTS

5-6 medium tomatoes, quartered

400 grams skinless and boneless chicken breasts

2 inches ginger

5-6 garlic cloves

2 green chillies, roughly chopped

¼ cup fresh coriander, roughly chopped

Salt to taste

1 medium onion, roughly sliced

1 teaspoon red chilli powder

2 teaspoons coriander powder

1 teaspoon cumin powder

1 teaspoon oil

½ teaspoon mustard seeds

8-10 curry leaves

2 teaspoons rice flour

½ teaspoon garam masala powder

METHOD

- Roughly cut chicken into small pieces. Grind ginger and garlic to a fine paste.
- Mince chicken along with green chillies, half the chopped coriander and salt to a smooth, fine mixture.
- Divide the mixture into sixteen equal portions, shape into balls and refrigerate until required.

- In a pressure cooker, combine the tomatoes, onion, ginger-garlic paste, remaining chopped coriander, chilli powder, coriander powder, cumin powder, salt and one cup of water, and cook under pressure for five or six minutes.
- Turn off the heat and let the mixture rest for fifteen minutes. Remove the lid and cool the contents to room temperature. Blend the mixture to a fine purée.
- Heat oil in non-stick pan; add mustard seeds and when they start to splutter, add curry leaves. Stir-fry for a few seconds.
- Stir in the puréed tomato mixture and one cup of water and bring to a boil.
- Reduce heat and gently slide in the prepared chicken balls. Cover the pan with a tight-fitting lid and simmer for fifteen minutes.
- Mix rice flour in one-fourth cup of water and add to the gravy, stirring gently to mix. Simmer for five minutes and add garam masala powder.
- Serve hot.

Diet Plans: A C

Portion: 1 bowl (1½ katori) with 4 chicken kofta

Chettinaad Grilled Chicken

INGREDIENTS

1 whole (600 grams) chicken

1 medium onion, roughly chopped

½ inch ginger, roughly chopped

2-3 garlic cloves, roughly chopped

2 green chillies, roughly chopped

2-3 dried red chillies

½ teaspoon turmeric powder

1 tablespoon lemon juice

2 tablespoons rice flour

Salt to taste

10-12 curry leaves, finely sliced

4 teaspoons oil

METHOD

- Slit the chicken through the backbone and the breast, into two equal halves. Make three to four half-inch deep cuts on breast and leg pieces.
- Grind together the onions, ginger, garlic, green chillies and dried red chillies to a fine paste, adding a little water if required.
- Blend the turmeric powder, lemon juice and rice flour into the prepared paste and mix in the salt.
- Apply the paste thoroughly and liberally over the chicken pieces and leave to marinate for two to three hours,

preferably in the refrigerator. Add the curry leaves to the chicken and mix.

- Heat oil in a non-stick grill pan; add the marinated chicken and sauté for two minutes on each side to seal in the juices.
- Reduce the heat to medium, cover and cook for fifteen to twenty minutes, turning over and basting frequently with the remaining marinade. Sprinkle a little water if the chicken begins to dry out.
- When almost done, increase the heat to high and cook until the chicken is crisp and golden.
- Cut into smaller pieces and serve hot.

Diet Plans: A C

Portion: 6–8 pieces chicken

Spiced Chicken Bites

INGREDIENTS

400 grams skinless, boneless chicken, cut into ½-inch pieces

2 teaspoons cumin seeds

1 tablespoon coriander seeds

10 black peppercorns

3-4 cloves

1 inch cinnamon

1 medium onion, roughly sliced

1 inch ginger, roughly sliced

4 garlic cloves

3-4 green chillies, halved

1 tablespoon lemon juice

Salt to taste

2 teaspoons oil

METHOD

- Dry-roast cumin seeds, coriander seeds, peppercorns, cloves and cinnamon.
- Mix together the roasted spices, onion, ginger, garlic, green chillies and lemon juice and grind to a fine paste. Add salt and mix well.
- Marinate chicken in the spice paste, preferably in the refrigerator, for two hours.
- Heat oil in a non-stick pan; add the marinated chicken and cook on medium heat for five minutes, stirring continuously.
- Reduce heat, cover and cook on low heat for five minutes, or until the chicken is tender, stirring occasionally. Serve hot.

Diet Plans: A C

Portion: 6-8 pieces chicken

Rajasthani Pulao with Chana Dal

INGREDIENTS

1½ cups rice, soaked for 2 hours and drained

¼ cup split Bengal gram, (chana dal), soaked for 2 hours and drained

2 teaspoons oil

1 inch cinnamon

2 cloves

2 green cardamoms

1 black cardamom

1 bay leaf (tej pata)

1 teaspoon cumin seeds

5-6 black peppercorns

3 teaspoons red chilli powder

½ teaspoon turmeric powder

1½ teaspoons coriander powder

Salt to taste

1½ tablespoons dried mint leaves

METHOD

- Heat the oil in a deep non-stick pan; add the cinnamon, cloves, cardamoms, bay leaf, cumin seeds and peppercorns, and sauté for one minute.
- Add the chilli powder, turmeric powder, coriander powder and salt. Cook for a few seconds and add the Bengal gram. Sauté for half a minute.
- Add three cups of water and bring to a boil. Stir in the dried mint leaves.
- Add the rice and stir to mix. Cover the pan and cook until the rice is tender. Serve hot.

Diet Plans: A B

Portion: 1 bowl (1½ katori)

Mushroom Quinoa Risotto

INGREDIENTS

½ cup quartered button mushrooms

½ cup quinoa, soaked

2 tablespoons brown rice, soaked

1 teaspoon olive oil

1 medium onion, finely chopped

1 teaspoon finely chopped garlic

3 cups Vegetable Stock (page 307)

Salt to taste

Crushed black peppercorns to taste

2 teaspoons grated processed cheese (optional)

METHOD

- Heat the olive oil in a deep non-stick pan.
- Add the chopped onion and sauté until translucent. Add the garlic and sauté for half a minute.
- Add the button mushrooms and quinoa and mix well.
- Add the brown rice and two cups vegetable stock and stir to mix. Cook for five to seven minutes. Add the remaining vegetable stock, salt and crushed peppercorns, and cook until the quinoa and rice are done.
- Add the grated cheese and mix well. Cook until the water reduces to half and the mixture is creamy.
- Transfer to a serving platter and serve immediately.

Diet Plans: A B

Portion: 1 cup (1 katori)

Gehun ki Khichdi

INGREDIENTS

1 cup broken wheat (lapsi)

2 teaspoons oil

1 teaspoon cumin seeds

A pinch of asafoetida (hing)

½ medium carrot, cut into ½-inch pieces

5 French beans, cut into ½-inch pieces

1 small potato, cut into ½-inch pieces

1 medium tomato, chopped

Salt to taste

1 tablespoon chopped fresh coriander

METHOD

- Soak the broken wheat in one and a half cups of water for half an hour. Drain and set aside.
- Heat the oil in a pressure cooker; add the cumin seeds and when they begin to change colour, add the asafoetida, carrot, French beans, potato and tomatoes. Sauté for a minute.
- Add the drained wheat and sauté for three or four minutes. Add two and a half cups of water and salt. Seal the cooker with the lid and cook over medium heat until the pressure is released twice (two whistles). Lower the heat and cook for another two or three minutes.
- Remove the lid when the pressure has reduced completely. Serve, garnished with chopped coriander.

Diet Plans: A B

Portion: 1 bowl (1½ katori)

Ragi Panki

INGREDIENTS

1½ cups finger millet flour (ragi), sifted

¼ cup whole-wheat flour (atta), sifted

4 tablespoons low-fat yogurt, whisked

1½ teaspoons finely chopped green chilli

½ teaspoon finely chopped ginger

2 teaspoons cumin seeds, roasted and crushed

2 pinches of soda bicarbonate

5-6 banana leaves, cut into 16 (6 inches) squares

Spray oil for greasing

METHOD

- Combine the two types of flour in a bowl; stir in the yogurt and three cups of water.
- Add the chilli, ginger and crushed cumin seeds and mix. Adjust the consistency by adding more water, if necessary, to make a batter of pouring consistency. Stir in the soda bicarbonate.
- Lightly grease the banana leaf squares with oil.
- Heat a non-stick tawa, and spray a little oil on it.
- Pour a small ladleful of batter on a banana leaf square and place it on the hot tawa.

- Cover with another banana leaf (oiled side down) and cook until tiny brown specks appear on the bottom leaf. Flip the panki and cook the other side.
- Alternatively, you can make a half-moon-shaped panki by spreading the batter on one half of the leaf and folding the other side over.
- Cook the rest of the panki in the same way and serve in the leaves with Green Chutney (page 307) on the side.

Diet Plans: A B
Portion: 2-3 panki

Vegetable Thepla

INGREDIENTS

¾ cup whole-wheat flour (atta)

¼ cup gram flour (besan)

¼ cup chopped fresh fenugreek (methi)

1 medium carrot, grated

¼ medium cabbage, grated

1 tablespoon chopped fresh coriander

Salt to taste

¼ teaspoon red chilli powder

¼ teaspoon turmeric powder

½ teaspoon ginger-green chilli paste

3 teaspoons oil

Low-fat yogurt, as required

METHOD

- Mix together the two types of flour with the chopped fenugreek, carrot, cabbage, chopped coriander, salt, chilli powder, turmeric powder, ginger-green chilli paste and one teaspoon of oil.
- Add enough yogurt to make a semi-soft dough.
- Divide the dough into twelve equal portions and roll out each portion into a thin thepla.
- Heat a non-stick tawa and roast each thepla, drizzling a little oil all around the edges, until both sides are evenly cooked. Serve with chutney or fresh yogurt.

Chef's Tip

These thepla will last for a minimum of three days as no water is used to make the dough.

Diet Plans: A B

Portion: 2 thepla

Soya Parantha

INGREDIENTS

½ cup soya granules, powdered

1 cup whole-wheat flour (atta)

Salt to taste

1 green chilli, finely chopped

½ teaspoon carom seeds (ajwain)

½ teaspoon dried pomegranate seeds (anardana), crushed

1 tablespoon chopped fresh coriander

3 teaspoons oil

METHOD

- Place the soya granule powder in a bowl.
- Add the flour, salt, green chilli, carom seeds, pomegranate seeds, chopped coriander and one teaspoon oil, and mix well.
- Add half a cup of water and knead into a stiff dough. Cover with a damp cloth and allow it to rest for about fifteen minutes.
- Divide the dough into four equal portions, shape into balls, lightly dust each with a little flour and roll out into a thick parantha about five-inches in diameter.
- Heat a non-stick tawa on medium heat; place a parantha on it and cook for two to three minutes. Turn it over and cook the other side for two to three minutes.
- Brush a little oil on both sides and cook, pressing with a flat spoon, until both sides are light golden brown.
- Serve hot.

Diet Plans: A B

Portion: 1 parantha

Pyaaz aur Pudine ki Roti

INGREDIENTS

2 medium onions, finely chopped

1 cup finely chopped fresh mint

2 cups whole-wheat flour (atta)

Salt to taste

2 green chillies, chopped

½ teaspoon carom seeds (ajwain)

1 teaspoon dried pomegranate seeds (anardana), roasted and crushed

2 teaspoons oil

METHOD

- Place the flour and salt in a deep bowl.
- Add the onions, mint leaves, green chillies, carom seeds and dried pomegranate seeds and knead with sufficient water into a stiff dough.
- Cover with a damp cloth and leave it to rest for twenty to twenty-five minutes.
- Divide the dough into eight equal portions. Shape them into balls and roll out each one into a medium-sized roti.
- Heat a non-stick tawa; place one roti at a time on it, and cook for half a minute.
- Flip it over, brush with a little oil and turn it over again. Brush the other side with a little oil and cook, turning, until both sides are light golden brown. Serve hot.

Diet Plans: A B

Portion: 2 roti

Palak Parantha

INGREDIENTS

1 bunch (250 grams) spinach leaves (palak)

1 cup whole-wheat flour (atta)

2 green chilli, seeded and chopped

Salt to taste

3 teaspoons ghee + for cooking

METHOD

- Chop a few spinach leaves and set aside. Blanch the rest and refresh in cold water.
- Purée the blanched spinach leaves and green chilli together.
- Sift the flour with salt and make a soft dough with the spinach purée, chopped spinach and water if needed. Cover with a damp cloth and set aside for thirty minutes.
- Divide the dough into six equal portions and shape into balls. Roll out each portion, spread some ghee and fold in half. Fold again into quarter. Roll out into six-inch triangles.
- Heat a non-stick tawa; place a parantha on it and cook for two to three minutes. Turn it over and brush with a little oil. Turn again and brush lightly with oil. Cook until both sides are evenly cooked.
- Serve hot with low-fat yogurt.

Diet Plans: A B

Portion: 1½ paranthe

Bajra Methi na Dhebra

INGREDIENTS

½ cup pearl millet (bajra) flour

½ cup chopped fresh fenugreek leaves (methi)

1 tablespoon gram flour (besan)

¼ teaspoon asafoetida (hing)

Salt to taste

1 teaspoon ginger paste

1 tablespoon chopped green chillies

1 teaspoon red chilli powder

2 tablespoons low-fat yogurt

2 teaspoons oil

METHOD

- Combine the millet flour, fenugreek leaves, gram flour, asafoetida, salt, ginger paste, green chillies, chilli powder and yogurt in a bowl. Add enough water and knead into a semi-stiff dough.
- Heat a non-stick tawa.
- Grease your palms with oil; divide dough into six equal portions and roll into balls. Pat each ball between your palms into small, thick roti.
- Place on the hot tawa and cook, flipping it over, until evenly cooked on both sides. Serve hot.

Diet Plans: A B

Portion: 1½ dhebra

Ragi aur Tofu Parantha

INGREDIENTS

Parantha

¾ cup finger millet (ragi) flour

¼ cup whole-wheat flour

½ teaspoon white sesame seeds

2 teaspoons ghee

Stuffing

½ cup grated bean curd (tofu)

2 green chillies, chopped

1 tablespoon chopped fresh coriander

1 small onion, chopped

1½ teaspoons chaat masala

Salt to taste

METHOD

- Mix together sesame seeds and both types of flour and knead with enough water to make a soft dough. Cover with a damp cloth and leave to rest for half an hour.
- To make the stuffing, combine the tofu, green chillies, chopped coriander, onion, chaat masala and salt in a bowl, and mix well. Divide the stuffing into four equal portions. Divide the dough into four equal portions, shape into balls and press between your palms.
- Roll out each portion of the dough into a four-inch disc that is thinner at the edges. Place a portion of the stuffing in the centre, gather the edges together, shape into a ball and roll out into a seven-inch round parantha.
- Heat a non-stick tawa. Place each parantha on it and cook, turning it over once, and drizzle a few drops of ghee around it. Turn it over again and spread a little ghee on the other side. Cook until both sides are cooked. Serve.

Diet Plans: A B

Portion: 1 parantha

Chicken Keema Parantha

INGREDIENTS

Parantha

1 cup whole-wheat flour (atta)

Salt to taste

2 teaspoons oil (optional)

Stuffing

125 grams minced chicken (keema)

½ cup low-fat yogurt

Salt to taste

½ tablespoon ginger-garlic paste

1 green chilli, chopped

1 tablespoon oil

1 teaspoon cumin seeds

1 medium onion, chopped

½ tablespoon red chilli powder

½ tablespoon coriander powder

½ teaspoon garam masala powder

1 tablespoon chopped fresh coriander

METHOD

- To make the parantha dough, sift the flour with salt in a deep bowl.
- Add sufficient water and knead into a stiff dough.
- Divide the dough into four equal portions and roll into balls.
- Cover with a damp cloth and set aside for fifteen minutes.

- To make the stuffing, combine the minced chicken, yogurt, salt, ginger-garlic paste and green chilli in a bowl. Marinate in the refrigerator for at least an hour.
- Heat one tablespoon oil in a non-stick pan. Add the cumin seeds and when they begin to change colour, add the onion and sauté until translucent.
- Add the chilli powder and coriander powder and sauté for half a minute. Add the marinated minced chicken and cook on medium heat, stirring occasionally, until tender and dry.
- Remove from heat and add the garam masala powder and chopped coriander and mix. Set aside to cool. Divide into four equal portions.
- Flatten each ball of dough and place one portion of the cooked mince in the centre. Gather the edges together and press to seal well. Shape into a round ball. Roll out each ball into a six-inch disc.
- Heat a non-stick tawa and place a parantha on it and cook for a minute. Brush with a little oil. Flip the parantha over and cook for a minute, brushing lightly with oil. Cook until both sides are golden brown. Serve hot.

Diet Plan: A
Portion: 1 parantha

Chicken Hakka Noodles

INGREDIENTS

300 grams whole-wheat noodles

½ cup boneless chicken, boiled and shredded

2 teaspoons oil

1 medium onion, sliced

1 medium carrot, grated

1 medium green capsicum, cut into thin strips

¼ small cabbage, shredded

1 tablespoon light soy sauce

Salt to taste

¼ teaspoon white pepper powder

1 cup bean sprouts

1 stalk spring onion greens, finely chopped

METHOD

- Boil noodles in plenty of water until al dente (cooked, but still firm to the bite). Drain, refresh in cold water, drain again and spread on a plate to cool.
- Heat oil in a non-stick wok; add onion and stir-fry for a few seconds. Add carrot, capsicum and cabbage and stir-fry for two minutes, stirring and tossing continuously.
- Add chicken and stir-fry for one minute.
- Add noodles, soy sauce, salt and white pepper powder, and cook on high heat for a couple of minutes, or until the noodles are heated through, tossing continuously.
- Add bean sprouts, mix well and serve hot, garnished with spring onion greens.

Diet Plan: A

Portion: 1 bowl (1½ katori)

Five-Spice Noodles and Vegetable Stir-Fry

INGREDIENTS

1 teaspoon Chinese Five-Spice Powder (page 235)

200 grams whole-wheat noodles, boiled

1 medium carrot, sliced

7-8 fresh button mushrooms, sliced

8-10 broccoli florets

8-10 French beans, cut diagonally into small pieces

1 tablespoon cornflour

½ cup fresh orange juice

2 teaspoons oil

5-6 garlic cloves, chopped

1 medium onion, sliced

Salt to taste

2 teaspoons light soy sauce

1 teaspoon crushed red chillies

METHOD

- Mix the cornflour with orange juice in a bowl and set aside.
- Heat oil in a non-stick wok; add the garlic, carrot and mushrooms and stir-fry for thirty seconds.
- Add the onion, broccoli, French beans, salt, soy sauce, one-fourth teaspoon crushed chillies and five-spice powder and continue to stir-fry for three to four minutes.
- Add the cornflour-orange juice mixture and one cup of water. Stir and cook until the mixture thickens.
- Add the noodles and toss well to mix. Serve hot, garnished with remaining crushed red chillies.

Diet Plan: A

Portion: 1 bowl (1½ katori)

Gourmet Pasta

INGREDIENTS

Pasta

2 cups whole-wheat flour (atta)

2 tablespoons refined flour (maida)

1 teaspoon salt

2 teaspoons olive oil

2 egg whites

Sauce

6 medium tomatoes

2 teaspoons olive oil

1 medium onion, finely chopped

3-4 garlic cloves, finely chopped

1 teaspoon red chilli flakes

5-6 fresh basil leaves (tulsi), shredded

1 teaspoon crushed black peppercorns

Salt to taste

METHOD

- For the pasta, sieve both the flours together.
- Add salt, one teaspoon oil and the egg whites, one by one. Sprinkle water and knead into a soft dough.
- Rest the dough, covered with a damp cloth, for thirty minutes.
- Knead the dough well once again. Sprinkle dry flour and roll the dough into as thin a sheet as possible. Trim the sides to form a rectangle. Sprinkle dry flour liberally and roll it up tightly.
- With a sharp knife cut the roll into half to three-fourth centimeter thick portions. Open out the rolls and spread out on a mesh and let them dry in a cool airy place overnight.

- To make the sauce, blanch the tomatoes for two minutes in boiling water. Drain, peel, remove seeds and chop roughly.
- Heat oil in a non-stick pan; add onion and garlic and sauté until onions turn translucent. Add red chilli flakes and toss well. Add the basil, reserving some for garnishing.
- Add the tomatoes and cook until the mixture starts bubbling. Add the crushed peppercorns and salt and mix well.
- While the sauce is cooking, boil plenty of water, adding one teaspoon oil and salt. Add the pasta to the boiling water and stir. Cook until it is just done or al dente (cooked, but still firm to the bite). Pour in one cup cold water and drain the pasta well.
- Add the cooked pasta to the sauce and toss over high heat until heated through. Adjust seasoning and serve hot, garnished with the reserved basil.

Chef's Tip

You can also make the pasta in a pasta machine. The method of preparing the dough will remain the same.

But, if you are short of time, you can use 3 cups cooked whole-wheat pasta for this recipe.

Diet Plans: A B

Portion: 1 bowl (1½ katori)

Pasta with Chicken and Cherry Tomatoes

INGREDIENTS

3 cups cooked whole-wheat short pasta

200 grams boneless chicken, cut into thin strips

12 cherry tomatoes, halved

1 teaspoon olive oil

8-10 garlic cloves, chopped

1 teaspoon red chilli flakes

1 sprig fresh thyme or 1 teaspoon dried thyme

4 fresh button mushrooms, thickly sliced

Salt to taste

¼ teaspoon crushed black peppercorns

1 cup skimmed milk

1 tablespoon chopped fresh parsley

METHOD

- Heat the olive oil in a non-stick pan; add the garlic and sauté until golden brown.
- Add the chilli flakes, chicken and thyme and sauté on high heat for two to three minutes.
- Add the cherry tomatoes and mushrooms and cook for two to three minutes.
- Add the pasta and toss well. Add the salt, crushed peppercorns and milk and mix well. Cook until heated through.
- Serve hot, garnished with the chopped parsley.

Diet Plan: A

Portion: 1 bowl (1½ katori)

Arbi ki Kadhi

INGREDIENTS

250 grams colocasia tubers (arbi), boiled

¼ cup water chestnut flour (singhare ka atta)

1½ cups sour low-fat yogurt

Rock salt (sendha namak) to taste

1 teaspoon red chilli powder

½ teaspoon turmeric powder

1 teaspoon oil

½ teaspoon cumin seeds

2-3 dried red chillies, broken into large bits

1 tablespoon chopped fresh coriander

METHOD

- Cool the colocasia slightly, peel and cut into half-inch thick slices.
- Whisk the water chestnut flour into the yogurt until smooth.
- Add the rock salt, chilli powder and turmeric powder and mix again. Add two cups of water and whisk well.
- Heat one teaspoon oil in a deep non-stick pan; add the cumin seeds and red chillies. When the cumin seeds begin to change colour, stir in the yogurt mixture. Cook for five minutes, stirring continuously.
- Add the boiled colocasia and mix. Continue cooking for five more minutes or until the kadhi is of the desired consistency. Garnish with chopped coriander and serve hot.

Diet Plans: A B

Portion: 1 bowl (1½ katori)

Dal Mizaaz

INGREDIENTS

¾ cup skinless split green gram (dhuli moong dal), soaked for ½ hour

¼ cup split pigeon peas (arhar dal/toovar dal), soaked for ½ hour

½ teaspoon turmeric powder

Salt to taste

2 teaspoons oil

½ tablespoon cumin seeds

1 small onion, chopped

1 small tomato, chopped

15 garlic cloves, chopped

1 inch ginger, cut into thin strips

½ tablespoon coriander powder

½ tablespoon cumin powder

¼ tablespoon garam masala powder

½ tablespoon red chilli powder

METHOD

- Drain and cook the green gram and pigeon peas with two and a half cups of water, turmeric powder and salt in a pressure cooker until pressure is released five to six times (five to six whistles).
- Heat one teaspoon oil in a deep non-stick pan. Add the cumin seeds and sauté until fragrant. Add onion and sauté until light brown.
- Add the tomato and sauté until soft. Add the garlic and continue to sauté for a minute.

¾ cup chopped fresh mint leaves

¼ cup chopped fresh coriander

½ tablespoon lemon juice

For garnish

A sprig of fresh coriander leaves

A sprig of fresh mint leaves

- Add the ginger strips and sauté for a minute.
- Add the coriander powder, cumin powder, garam masala powder, chilli powder, one-fourth cup mint leaves and sauté for two minutes.
- Add the dals, the remaining mint leaves and chopped coriander and mix well.
- When the mixture comes to a boil, add salt, the remaining oil and one-fourth cup of water. Stir in the lemon juice and mix well.
- Serve hot, garnished with fresh coriander and mint sprigs.

Diet Plans: A B C
Portion: 1 bowl (1½ katori)

Sprouted Hara Chana Amti

INGREDIENTS

1 cup green Bengal gram (hara chana)

1½ teaspoons oil

¼ teaspoon asafoetida (hing)

¼ teaspoon mustard seeds

2 dried red chillies, broken in half

3-4 garlic cloves, finely chopped

2-3 green chillies, finely chopped

2 tablespoons Tamarind Pulp (page 307)

½ teaspoon turmeric powder

Salt to taste

1 teaspoon grated jaggery

¼ teaspoon carom seeds (ajwain), crushed

METHOD

- Wash the gram two or three times, and soak in plenty of water for four to five hours.
- Drain, tie in a moist piece of muslin and leave in a warm place for two days or until the gram sprouts. Make sure that the cloth is always moist.

- Heat oil in a non-stick pan; add asafoetida and mustard seeds and when they splutter, add red chillies and sauté for half a minute.
- Add garlic and green chillies and stir-fry for half a minute.
- Dilute the tamarind pulp with three cups of water and add to the pan.
- Sprinkle turmeric powder, salt and jaggery and stir over high heat; cook until the jaggery dissolves.
- Add the sprouted gram and the crushed carom seeds and stir to mix thoroughly.
- Cover and cook for ten to fifteen minutes on medium heat. Serve hot.

Diet Plans: A B C
Portion: 1 bowl (1½ katori)

Dal Khilma

INGREDIENTS

1½ cups skinless split green gram (dhuli moong dal)

3 inches ginger

3 green chillies, chopped

3 teaspoons oil

A pinch asafoetida (hing)

1 teaspoon cumin seeds

¼ teaspoon turmeric powder

½ teaspoon red chilli powder

Salt to taste

½ teaspoon garam masala powder

1 tablespoon lemon juice

2 tablespoons chopped fresh coriander

METHOD

- Chop half the ginger and cut the remaining into thin strips.
- Cook the green gram with green chillies and chopped ginger in three cups of water until just done, ensuring that the grains remain separate.
- Heat oil in a non-stick kadai; add asafoetida and cumin seeds. When the cumin seeds begin to change colour, add turmeric powder and sauté for half a minute.
- Add the cooked dal, chilli powder and salt and stir gently to mix. Cook on low heat for two to three minutes taking care not to mash the dal.
- Sprinkle garam masala powder and lemon juice. Garnish with chopped coriander and ginger strips and serve hot.

Diet Plans: A B C

Portion: 1 bowl (1½ katori)

Drumstick Dal

INGREDIENTS

4 large drumsticks, fibrous strings removed and cut into four pieces

8 teaspoons split pigeon peas (toor dal), soaked for 1 hour

A pinch of asafoetida (hing)

½ teaspoon turmeric powder

A pinch of salt

1 teaspoon chopped garlic

1 teaspoon red chilli powder

2 teaspoons coriander-cumin powder

1 teaspoon Tamarind Pulp (page 307)

METHOD

- Pressure-cook the pigeon peas with asafoetida and a pinch of turmeric powder in one and a half cups of water until the pressure is released four times (four whistles).
- Boil the drumstick pieces with salt and sufficient water until soft. Drain and set aside. Dry-roast the garlic in a non-stick pan for two minutes. Add the remaining turmeric powder, chilli powder, coriander-cumin powder and tamarind pulp, mix well and cook for a few minutes.
- Add the pigeon peas and drumsticks, stir to mix and cook for three to four minutes. Serve hot.

Recipe courtesy Dr Sarita Davare

Diet Plans: A B C

Portion: 1 bowl (1½ katori)

Doodhi Chana Dal

INGREDIENTS

1 small (500 grams) bottle gourd (doodhi/lauki), cut into 1-inch pieces

½ cup split Bengal gram (chana dal), soaked for 1 hour

Salt to taste

½ teaspoon turmeric powder

½ teaspoon red chilli powder

2 teaspoons coriander powder

2 green chillies, chopped

½ inch ginger, chopped

2 teaspoons ghee

½ teaspoon cumin seeds

A large pinch asafoetida (hing)

½ teaspoon sugar

2 teaspoons lemon juice

2 tablespoons chopped fresh coriander

METHOD

- Drain and transfer the split Bengal gram into a non-stick pan.
- Add the bottle gourd, salt, turmeric powder, chilli powder, coriander powder, green chillies, ginger and two cups of water, and bring to a boil on high heat.

- Reduce the heat, cover and cook for twenty minutes or until the gram is soft and the gourd is cooked. Mash slightly using the back of a ladle and mix well. Transfer to a bowl and set aside.
- Heat ghee in a non-stick pan on medium heat. Add the cumin seeds and asafoetida and sauté until the seeds change colour.
- Add the cooked mixture and stir. Add the sugar and stir to mix. Simmer for two minutes, stirring occasionally. Add the lemon juice and stir.
- Garnish with the chopped coriander and serve immediately.

Diet Plans: A B C

Portion: 1 bowl (1½ katori)

Microwave Ankurit Moong Kadhi

INGREDIENTS

¾ cup sprouted whole green gram (ankurit moong)

1 cup low-fat yogurt

¼ cup gram flour (besan)

1 teaspoon grated jaggery

1 inch ginger, chopped

Salt to taste

2 teaspoons oil

4 dried red chillies, broken into 2 pieces

6-8 black peppercorns, crushed

½ teaspoon fenugreek seeds (methi dana)

½ teaspoon cumin seeds

7-8 curry leaves

¼ teaspoon asafoetida (hing)

METHOD

- Place sprouted green gram with two cups of water in a microwave-safe bowl. Cover and cook on MEDIUM for eight minutes. Drain any excess water.
- Whisk together yogurt and gram flour until smooth.
- Add two cups of water and mix well. Add jaggery and ginger and mix.

- Pour the mixture into a deep microwave-safe bowl and cook, covered, on HIGH for ten minutes, stirring once after five minutes. The mixture should have a moderately thick consistency.
- Add salt, cooked green gram and cook again on HIGH for five minutes.
- Put oil in a separate small microwave-safe bowl. Add red chillies, peppercorns, fenugreek seeds, cumin seeds, curry leaves and asafoetida.
- Cook, uncovered, on HIGH for two minutes. Remove and add to the kadhi. Serve hot.

Recipe courtesy Dr Sarita Davare

Diet Plans: A B C

Portion: 1 bowl (1½ katori)

Methi Varan

INGREDIENTS

3 cups finely chopped fresh fenugreek (methi)

4 cups Dal Stock (see Note below)

4 curry leaves

2 garlic cloves, chopped

½ teaspoon turmeric powder

1 teaspoon red chilli powder

½ teaspoon coriander-cumin powder

½ teaspoon salt

METHOD

- Dry-roast the curry leaves with garlic for a minute.
- Add the fenugreek and dal stock and stir to mix. Add the turmeric powder, chilli powder, coriander-cumin powder and salt. Mix well and bring to a boil.
- Serve hot.

Note: *Dal stock is the liquid strained after boiling dal.*

Recipe courtesy Dr Sarita Davare

Diet Plans: A B C

Portion: 1 bowl (1½ katori)

Kadi Patta Chutney

INGREDIENTS

2 cups curry leaves (kadi patta)

¼ cup roasted split Bengal gram

20-25 black peppercorns

Marble-sized ball of tamarind

Salt to taste

METHOD

- Roast the curry leaves, gram, peppercorns and tamarind separately until dry and crisp. Mix well. Set aside to cool.
- Grind the roasted ingredients to a powder.
- Add salt and mix well. Cool completely and store in an airtight container.

Diet Plans: A B C
Portion: 2-3 teaspoons

Daalia Chutney

INGREDIENTS

¾ cup roasted split Bengal gram (daalia)

1 green chilli, chopped

Salt to taste

½ teaspoon cumin seeds

1 cup low-fat yogurt

1 teaspoon oil

¼ teaspoon mustard seeds

1 dried red chilli, broken into bits

5-6 curry leaves

¼ teaspoon turmeric powder

METHOD

- Grind together roasted gram, green chilli, salt and cumin seeds in a blender.
- Transfer the mixture to a bowl. Add the yogurt and mix well.
- Heat the oil in a non-stick pan. Add the mustard seeds, red chilli, curry leaves and turmeric powder and sauté until the seeds splutter.
- Add the seasoning to the chutney and mix well.

Diet Plans: A B C
Portion: 2-3 tablespoons

Pickled Cucumbers

INGREDIENTS

4 small cucumbers

2 tablespoons white vinegar

1 teaspoon caster sugar or equivalent sugar substitute

1 teaspoon sesame (til) oil

Salt to taste

1 fresh red chilli, halved

METHOD

- Wash and halve unpeeled cucumbers.
- Remove seeds and cut into one-fourth-inch thick sticks.
- Heat vinegar, sugar and sesame oil in a non-stick pan.
- When the mixture comes to a boil turn off the heat and add the cucumbers and salt and mix well.
- Add the fresh red chilli and toss well to mix.

Diet Plans: A B C
Portion: 6-8 sticks

Apple Basoondi

INGREDIENTS

2 medium (300 grams) apples

5 cups skimmed milk

4 teaspoons sugar

4 almonds

4 pistachios

A few drops of screw pine/ pandanus (kewra) water

METHOD

- Bring the milk to a boil in a thick-bottomed pan.
- Lower the heat, add the sugar and simmer for fifteen to twenty minutes until it thickens. Remove from heat and set aside to cool.
- Blanch the almonds and pistachios in boiling water for two to three minutes. Drain, peel and cut into slivers. Set aside.
- Peel and grate the apples and add to the cooled milk immediately to avoid oxidation. Stir in the slivered nuts and screw pine water.
- Serve chilled.

Diet Plans: A B C
Portion: ½ cup (1 small katori)

Fresh Fruit Yogurt

INGREDIENTS

1 apple

8-10 cherries, stoned

Lemon juice

2 cups low-fat yogurt

2 teaspoons sugar or equivalent sugar substitute

4-5 saffron threads

1 teaspoon raisins

3-4 walnut halves or blanched almonds, finely chopped

METHOD

- Wash, peel, core the apple and cut into half-inch cubes. Sprinkle with a little lemon juice to prevent oxidation.
- Combine apples and cherries and refrigerate until ready to serve.
- In a bowl, combine yogurt, sugar and saffron and whisk until sugar is completely dissolved.
- Just before serving, mix in fruit and serve chilled, garnished with raisins and walnuts.

Note: *You can use any combination of fruit and dried fruit.*

Diet Plans: A B C
Portion: 1 cup (1 katori)

Ginger and Oatmeal Halwa

INGREDIENTS

½ tablespoon dried ginger powder (saunth)

¼ cup oatmeal

½ tablespoon oatmeal flour

¼ cup whole-wheat grains

2 teaspoons cow's milk ghee

½ tablespoon whole-wheat flour (atta)

2 teaspoons sugar or equivalent sugar substitute

2 almonds, roasted and slivered

2 pistachios, roasted and slivered

METHOD

- Soak whole-wheat grains in two cups of water for eight to ten hours. Drain and crush in a mixer. If the wheat is too dry add a little water.
- Heat 1 teaspoon ghee in a non-stick pan and sauté crushed whole-wheat for five minutes.
- Add oatmeal flour and whole-wheat flour and sauté for another two to three minutes. Add oatmeal and continue to sauté. Add sugar and three cups of water and mix well. Add more water, if necessary, and cook until it thickens and attains the consistency of halwa.
- Drizzle the remaining teaspoon of ghee on top. Add slivered almonds, pistachios and dried ginger powder and mix. Serve hot.

Diet Plans: A B
Portion: ½ cup/1 small katori

Kakdi che Ghavan

INGREDIENTS

1 medium cucumber, grated

¾ cup whole-wheat flour (atta)

¼ cup rice flour

2 tablespoons grated jaggery

Salt to taste

2 teaspoons cow's milk ghee

METHOD

- Combine grated cucumber, flour, rice flour, jaggery and salt.
- Add sufficient water to make a batter of pouring consistency.
- Heat a non-stick tawa and grease with a little ghee.
- Pour one-fourth ladleful of batter on it and spread into a thin round.
- Flip and cook on both sides until golden brown.
- Repeat the same with remaining batter. Serve hot.

Diet Plans: A B
Portion: 1 ghavan

Chocolate Phirni

INGREDIENTS

5 tablespoons raw rice

1 litre skimmed milk

3 tablespoons cocoa powder

2 tablespoons milk powder

2 teaspoons sugar or equivalent sugar substitute

4-5 pistachios, blanched and sliced

METHOD

- Soak rice for half an hour and grind to a coarse paste.
- Mix cocoa in one-fourth cup of cold milk. Mix milk powder in one-fourth cup of warm milk.
- Bring the remaining milk to a boil in a non-stick pan. Add the cocoa and milk powder mixtures to the boiling milk; cook, stirring continuously.
- Stir in the rice paste and cook, stirring, until the mixture attains a thick consistency.
- Remove from heat and mix in sugar.
- Pour into an earthenware pot. Sprinkle pistachios and leave the phirni to cool. Serve chilled.

Diet Plans: A B
Portion: ¾ cup (¾ katori)

Moong Dal Halwa

INGREDIENTS

½ cup split skinless green gram (dhuli moong dal), soaked

2-3 teaspoons sugar or equivalent sugar substitute

A generous pinch of saffron

½ cup skimmed milk

1 teaspoon cow's milk ghee

2 tablespoons khoya/ mawa, crumbled

2-3 almonds, sliced

METHOD

- Drain and grind the green gram coarsely using very little water.
- Soak the saffron in hot milk.
- Heat ghee in a thick-bottomed non-stick pan; add the coarsely ground gram and sauté, stirring continuously, over low heat, until it turns golden brown. This needs time and patience. Do not rush through this step.
- Add the sugar and saffron-flavoured milk. Stir to mix thoroughly and cook until the halwa is of dropping consistency. Add mawa and cook until it dissolves.
- Serve hot garnished with almonds.

Chef's Tip

Add one tablespoon of gram flour to melted ghee before adding the ground gram. It helps in even cooking of the ground gram and also prevents formation of lumps during cooking.

Diet Plans: A B C
Portion: ¾ cup (¾ katori)

Oatmeal Bars with Custard

INGREDIENTS

1 cup oatmeal

¼ cup honey

2 tablespoons chopped cashew nuts

1 tablespoon raisins

2 teaspoons butter

½ teaspoon cinnamon powder

½ tablespoon powdered sugar

1 cup skimmed milk

1 tablespoon custard powder

METHOD

- Preheat oven to 180°C/350°F/Gas Mark 4.
- Place oatmeal, honey, cashew nuts, raisins, butter, cinnamon powder and powdered sugar in a bowl and mix well.
- Transfer the mixture to a 6 x 8-inch baking tin and press lightly. Place the tin in the preheated oven and bake for ten to fifteen minutes. Remove from the oven and cut into bars.
- In the meanwhile, pour milk into a non-stick pan. Add custard powder and whisk well. Cook the mixture on medium heat until the custard thickens. Remove from heat and set aside.
- Pour a little custard in each serving plate. Arrange a bar in the centre and serve immediately.

Diet Plans: A B

Portion: 2 bars with ¼ cup custard

Rawa Kesari

INGREDIENTS

½ cup semolina (sooji)

2 teaspoons cow's milk ghee

1½ cups low-fat milk

10-12 raisins

4-10 almonds, chopped

A few saffron threads, mixed in 1 tablespoon water

¼ teaspoon green cardamom powder

2 teaspoons sugar or equivalent sugar substitute

METHOD

- Heat ghee in a non-stick kadai; add semolina and roast until golden.
- Mix milk with one and a half cups of water and bring to a boil. Add the milk to the roasted semolina and cook until the mixture thickens.
- Add raisins, almonds, saffron, cardamom powder and sugar and mix well. Serve hot.

Diet Plans: A B
Portion: ½ cup (1 small katori)

Quinoa Pistachio Bars

INGREDIENTS

½ cup roasted quinoa

¼ cup crushed roasted pistachios

1 cup seedless dates

1 tablespoon honey

A pinch of salt

Oil for greasing

METHOD

- Coarsely grind the dates in a food processor and transfer to a bowl.
- Add the honey, quinoa, pistachios and salt and mix well.
- Grease a 4 x 6-inch shallow tray with a few drops of oil. Spread the date-quinoa mixture in it evenly. Refrigerate for one hour.
- Cut into one-inch thick pieces and serve.

Diet Plans: A B
Portion: 2 bars

Basic Recipes

Chicken Stock

Boil 200 grams chicken bones in water for 5 minutes. Drain and discard water. Boil blanched bones with a roughly chopped carrot, celery stalk, leek, 2-3 parsley stalks, 6-7 black peppercorns, 5-6 cloves, 1 bay leaf and 10 cups of water. Remove any scum which rises to the surface and replace it with more cold water. Simmer for at least 1 hour. Remove from heat, strain, cool and store in a refrigerator until further use.

Fish Stock

Boil 200 grams fish bones, head, skin (any unutilised portions of fish), 5 cups of water, 1 sliced onion, 1 large button mushroom, 2-3 inch celery stalk, 1 bay leaf and 4-6 black peppercorns in a large pan. Remove any scum which floats to the top and simmer for fifteen minutes. Strain and use immediately.

Green Chutney

Grind 5 cups mint leaves, 3 cups coriander leaves, 10 green chillies, 3 onions and 3 inches of ginger to a fine paste, adding a little water if required. Stir in 1 tablespoon lemon juice and salt.

Tamarind Pulp

Soak 75 grams tamarind in 100 ml warm water for 10-15 minutes. Grind to a smooth paste and strain to remove any fibres. Store in an airtight container in the refrigerator.

Vegetable Stock

Peel, wash and chop 1 onion, ½ medium carrot, 2-3 inch celery stalk and 2-3 garlic cloves. Place in a pan with 1 bay leaf, 5-6 peppercorns, 2-3 cloves and 5 cups of water and bring to a boil. Lower heat and simmer for 15 minutes and strain. Cool and store in a refrigerator until further use.

Glossary

English	Hindi
Almonds	Badam
Aloe vera	Dritkumari
Amaranth	Rajgira
Apricots	Khubani
Asafoetida	Hing
Ash gourd	Petha
Barley	Jau
Basil leaves	Tulsi ke patte
Bay leaf	Tej patta
Bean sprouts	Ankurit moong
Beetroot	Chukandar
Black salt	Kala namak
Bottle gourd	Doodhi
Broad beans	Papdi
Buttermilk	Chhaas
Cabbage	Bandh gobhi
Capsicum	Shimla mirch
Cardamoms, black	Badi elaichi
Cardamoms, green	Chhoti elaichi
Carom seeds	Ajwain
Carrots	Gajar
Cauliflower	Phool gobi
Celery	Ajmud
Chickpeas	Kabuli chana
Cinnamon	Dalchini
Cloves	Laung

English	**Hindi**
Colocasia tubers	Arbi
Coriander seeds	Sabut dhania
Coriander, fresh	Hara dhania
Cottage cheese	Paneer
Cumin seeds	Jeera
Curry leaves	Kadi patta
Dates	Khajoor
Dates, dried	Chuhare
Dill leaves	Suva bhaji
Dried mango powder	Amchur
Drumsticks	Saijan ki phalli/sing
Egg white	Ande ki safedi
Fennel	Saunf
Fenugreek leaves, dried	Kasuri methi
Fenugreek seeds	Methi dana
Field beans, split	Sem ki dal
Fig	Anjeer
French beans	Farsi
Ginger	Adrak
Gram, Bengal, greem	Hare chane
Gram, Bengal, split	Chana dal
Gram, Bengal, split roasted	Daalia
Gram, black, skinless split	Dhuli urad dal
Gram, brown	Matki/moth
Gram, flour	Besan
Gram, green, skinless split	Dhuli moong dal
Gram, green whole	Sabut moong
Grapefruit	Chakotra
Indian gooseberries	Amla

English	Hindi
Jaggery	Gur
Kidney beans, red	Rajma
Lady's fingers	Bhindi
Lemon	Nimboo
Lentils, red split	Masoor dal
Lettuce	Salad patta
Maize	Makai
Milk, skimmed	Malai rahit doodh
Millet, finger	Nachni
Millet, pearl	Bajra
Mint, fresh	Pudina ke taaze patte
Mushroom	Khumb/dhingri
Musk melon	Kharbooj
Mustard	Sarson/rai
Oats/Oatmeal	Jai
Olive	Jaitun
Orange	Santara
Papaya	Papita
Parsley	Ajmoda
Peanuts	Moongphali
Pear	Naspati
Peas, green	Taaze matar
Peppercorns	Kali mirch
Pigeon peas, fresh green	Taaze hare toovar
Pigeon peas, split	Toovar dal/arhar dal
Pineapple	Ananas
Pistachios	Pista
Plum	Aloo bukhara
Pomegranate seeds	Anar ke dana

English	Hindi
Prunes	Sukhe aloo bukhare
Pumpkin	Kaddu
Radish, white	Mooli
Raisins	Kishmish
Refined flour	Maida
Rice, beaten	Poha
Rock salt	Sendha namak
Saffron	Kesar
Screw pine/pandanus	Kewra
Semolina	Rawa/sooji
Sesame	Til
Soda bicarbonate	Khane ka soda
Sorghum	Jowar
Spinach	Palak
Spring Onions	Hara pyaaz
Tamarind	Imli
Turmeric powder	Haldi
Unripe green mango	Keri
Vinegar	Sirka
Walnut	Akhrot
Water chestnuts	Singhara
Watermelon	Tarbooj
Whole-wheat flour	Atta
Yogurt	Dahi

Height/Weight chart for Indian Men and Women*

Height in Metre and (Feet/inches)	Men (In Kgs)/Lbs	Women (In Kgs)/ Lbs
1.52 (5' 0")	---	50.8 to 54.4/112-120
1.54 (5' 1")	---	51.7 to 55.3/114-122
1.57 (5' 2")	56.3 to 60.3/124-133	53.1 to 56.7/117-125
1.60 (5' 3")	57.6 to 61.7/127-136	54.4 to 58.1/120-128
1.63 (5' 4")	58.9 to 63.5/130-140	56.3 to 59.9/124-132.
1.65 (5' 5")	60.8 to 65.3/134-44	57.6 to 61.2/127-135
1.68 (5' 6")	62.2 to 66.7/137-147	58.9 to 63.5/130-140
1.70 (5' 7")	64.0 to 68.5/141-151	60.8 to 65.3/134-144
1.73 (5' 8")	65.8 to 70.8/145-156	62.2 to 66.7/137-147
1.75 (5' 9")	67.6 to 72.6/149-160	64.0 to 68.5/141-151
1.78 (5'10")	69.4 to 74.4/153-164	65.8 to 70.3/145-155
1.80 (5'11")	71.2 to 76.2/157-168	67.1 to 71.7/148-158
1.83 (6' 0")	73.0 to 78.5/161-173	68.5 to 73.9/151-163
1.85 (6' 1")	75.3 to 80.7/166-178	---
1.88 (6'2")	77.6 to 83.5/171-184	---
1.90 (6' 3")	79.8 to 85.7/176-189	---

Special Note :

Upto age of 30 years. : 10% above standard is acceptable.

Between 30-35 years : Standard is optimum weight.

Above 35 years : 10% below standard is acceptable.

*As compiled by the LIC of India and accepted as standard weight chart all over India.